Stroke Rehabilitation
A Collaborative Approach

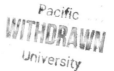

Edited by

Robert Fawcus

Consultant Speech and Language Therapist
Nuffield Hospital, Tunbridge Wells

Former Lecturer, Department of Medicine,
The United Medical and Dental Schools of St Thomas and Guy's
and
Professor of Clinical Communication Studies,
City University, London

Blackwell
Science

© 2000 by
Blackwell Science Ltd
Editorial Offices:
Osney Mead, Oxford OX2 0EL
25 John Street, London WC1N 2BL
23 Ainslie Place, Edinburgh EH3 6AJ
350 Main Street, Malden
  MA 02148 5018, USA
54 University Street, Carlton
  Victoria 3053, Australia
10, rue Casimir Delavigne
  75006 Paris, France

Other Editorial Offices:

Blackwell Wissenschafts-Verlag GmbH
Kurfürstendamm 57
10707 Berlin, Germany

Blackwell Science KK
MG Kodenmacho Building
7–10 Kodenmacho Nihombashi
Chuo-ku, Tokyo 104, Japan

The right of the Author to be identified as the
Author of this Work has been asserted in
accordance with the Copyright, Designs and
Patents Act 1988.

First published 2000

Set in 10/13pt Times
by DP Photosetting, Aylesbury, Bucks
Printed and bound in Great Britain by
The Alden Press, Oxford and Northampton

The Blackwell Science logo is a trade mark of
Blackwell Science Ltd, registered at the United
Kingdom Trade Marks Registry

DISTRIBUTORS

Marston Book Services Ltd
PO Box 269
Abingdon
Oxon OX14 4YN
(*Orders:* Tel: 01235 465500
            Fax: 01235 465555)

USA
Blackwell Science, Inc.
Commerce Place
350 Main Street
Malden, MA 02148 5018
(*Orders:* Tel: 800 759 6102
            781 388 8250
            Fax: 781 388 8255)

Canada
Login Brothers Book Company
324 Saulteaux Crescent
Winnipeg, Manitoba R3J 3T2
(*Orders:* Tel: 204 837 2987
            Fax: 204 837 3116)

Australia
Blackwell Science Pty Ltd
54 University Street
Carlton, Victoria 3053
(*Orders:* Tel: 03 9347 0300
            Fax: 03 9347 5001)

A catalogue record for this title is available
from the British Library

ISBN 0-632-04998-7

Library of Congress
Cataloging-in-Publication Data
Stroke rehabilitation: a collaborative approach/
  edited by Robert Fawcus.
      p. cm.
    Includes bibliographical references and
index.
    ISBN 0-632-04998-7 (pbk.)
    1. Cerebrovascular disease – Patients –
Rehabilitation.   2. Medical cooperation.
3. Health care teams.   4. Holistic medicine.
I. Fawcus, Robert.
[DNLM: 1. Cerebrovascular Disorders –
rehabilitation.   2. Patient Care Team.
WL 355 S92136 1999]
RC388.5.S85623   1999
616.8'1 – dc21
DNLM/DLC
for Library of Congress   99-32628
                                             CIP

For further information on
Blackwell Science, visit our website:
www.blackwell-science.com

Dedicated to

H.F.
M.A.F.
P.W.H.F.

and the patients and clients from whom
we have learnt so much

Contents

Contributors

Graham Boswell BA (Hons), BSc (Hons), MA Ed, RGN Lecturer in Neurological/Neurosurgical Nursing, City University, St Bartholomews School of Nursing and Midwifery, London

Shelagh Brumfitt PhD, MRCSLT Senior Lecturer in Language and Therapeutics, Department of Human Communication Sciences, University of Sheffield

Avril Drummond PhD, MSc, DipCOT Research Occupational Therapist, Ageing and Disability Research Unit, The Medical School, University of Nottingham

Robert Fawcus BSc, FRCSLT Formerly Professor of Clinical Communication Studies, City University, London, Consultant Speech and Language Therapist, Nuffield Hospital, Tunbridge Wells, Kent

Marion Hildick-Smith CBE, MA, MD, FRCP Consultant Geriatrician, Kent and Canterbury Hospital, Canterbury, Kent

Polly Laidler MCSP Consultant Neurophysiotherapist based in Essex, Clinical Specialist in Stroke Rehabilitation

Jane Marshall PhD, MRCSLT Research Speech and Language Therapist, Department of Language and Communication Science, City University, London

Simon B.N. Thompson PhD, PGDipIS, MPhil, BA (Hons), CPsychol, AFBPsS Consultant Clinical Neuropsychologist/Head of Clinical Psychology and Neuropsychology Services for Older Adults, Sussex Weald and Downs NHS Trust, Chichester, West Sussex

Preface

Any collaborative enterprise is heavily dependent upon the relationship which develops between the participants. The origins of the present work are derived from an idea proposed by Maggie Fawcus and fostered by her against considerable odds. The baton was handed to me after she had established the general structure of the book and engaged most of the contributors. Due to the idiosyncracies of professional fate, I had returned to working with dysphasic adults after years of activity in other areas.

Throughout our careers we have both been convinced of the necessity to approach the problems of dysphasic adults in a collaborative environment but, in common with many colleagues in whatever the discipline involved, we have not always found ourselves in a context where this is a practical possibility.

The book begins with a number of chapters outlining the medical background and approach to the difficulties of patients who have suffered a cerebrovascular accident or similar pathology which has, in some measure, affected their ability to walk, speak, read, write or continue a normal life. The term 'patient' is employed because this is the common parlance in such settings. In succeeding chapters the physical and social consequences of stroke are examined and some contributors prefer to use designations such as 'client'. At one stage some of us feared we would be forced to use the term customer!

When inviting people to any sort of party, there is always the problem of those who have been left out. The difficulty with the host of people involved in the care of an individual following a stroke is that contributions to the book from everyone would require a number of volumes. What we have attempted to convey are the principles of collaboration in different contexts which apply just as importantly to general practitioners, dentists, social workers, care staff and others who have not figured prominently in this work despite the major contribution which they can provide to the person recovering from a stroke.

Robert Fawcus

Chapter 1

A Collaborative Approach to Stroke Care

Robert Fawcus

The sudden loss of any capacity causes severe distress to both the individual affected and those in his or her immediate environment. Even a slight reduction of power in the upper dominant limb can severely disrupt skills such as writing, cooking or precision tool use. If this is accompanied by the limitation of mobility associated with a right hemiplegia, the catastrophic effects of stroke on an individual and his/her family, friends and working colleagues become immediately obvious.

The loss or disruption of language skills is, for most people, the most devastating result of a cerebrovascular accident. For the person struggling to come to terms with limitations in the ability to express him/herself, taken for granted only days before the stroke, the anger and distress is unmistakeable. When this is exacerbated by difficulties in understanding even simple utterances made by family, nursing staff and physicians, the levels of anxiety and frustration are overpowering. The anguish of close friends and family members is made far worse by their concerns about how they should best attempt to communicate with their stricken loved one.

This book is written for all those who are professionally involved in the management of stroke. Its aim is to provide a greater understanding of the problems to be faced and the strategies employed to overcome them. It will also help to give health care students and the newly qualified a broader perspective of stroke management and to facilitate the interdisciplinary cooperation which is essential if rehabilitation programmes are to be optimally effective.

The book brings together the experience and expertise of a group of health-care professionals who give their own perspective on the problems they encounter daily and the very specific skills involved in dealing with these problems. Inevitably, this means that there is some overlap between the chapters. For example, all members of the medical and rehabilitation team are concerned with the psychosocial aspect of stroke, and authors comment on its importance from their own perspective and describe their role in helping to deal with it.

It is essential that all members of a team, whether *ad hoc* or specifically organized for the purpose of rehabilitation, have clear lines of communication so that optimal benefit may be obtained from their input. In many hospital settings the team is loosely coordinated, but specific case conferences can be effective in determining aims and expectations. Often the hospital notes and the nursing record are the prime means by which information is conveyed, augmented by chance encounters in corridors or at the bedside. In a general hospital setting the 'team' may be drawn from an array of nursing groups and medical firms with no obvious cohesion. There are clearly considerable advantages to be gained from a recognized rehabilitation team which has developed agreed patterns of assessment and treatment.

The very name 'stroke' reflects the sudden and unexpected onset of this devastating condition which may lead to a completely different lifestyle for both patient and carer. Where spontaneous recovery takes place, these effects will fortunately be only temporary. When, however, the hemiplegia and communication difficulties persist, patients and their families face major and lasting changes in their social life, their financial circumstances and the roles they play within the family and at work. These changes will depend on a number of factors, including the severity of the stroke, the patient's age, and particular circumstances at the time of the stroke. In the case of an elderly patient who has retired from work, these changes may not be quite so dramatic, but caring for a physically disabled partner will impose a heavy burden on an ageing carer. The effects of the stroke may also prevent the patient from enjoying leisure activities which have given pleasure and meaning to his or her retirement.

The outlook for the patient with a left hemiplegia and no speech or language problems is often not as bleak as it would be for someone with both a right hemiplegia and aphasia. It may still make a return to work problematic if manual skills or the need to drive a car were involved. Whilst hemiplegic patients can and do learn to drive specially adapted cars, the risk of having a fit may prevent them from doing so for up to two years. This will add to the frustration of their immobility, since a dense hemiplegia often makes using public transport a hazardous activity. Whilst some stroke patients may return to work, the present employment situation makes it extremely difficult to find a suitable occupation. Some employers play a very responsible role in trying to re-integrate both hemiplegic and communication impaired employees into their old jobs. This requires providing support and making adjustments, but the results can be satisfactory for employer and employee alike.

The majority of patients and their families are totally unprepared for the onset of a stroke. Its suddenness, and the profound physical and psychological changes in the individual, can lead to serious problems of adjustment for both patient and family. These difficulties are often compounded by a lack of adequate information and support from some of the professionals involved in the early management of stroke. This is even more likely to occur if the patient is not admitted to hospital. Fortunately, this is not always the case, and the past decade has seen the development of stroke units which recognize and try to meet the needs of both carers and patients.

Not only may the family be facing a vastly changed lifestyle because of loss of income, but they may also have serious financial worries, such as inability to keep up mortgage payments. All this may exacerbate the typical pattern of post-stroke depression which, in its turn, tends to erode the patient's motivation and confidence. It is very important that the family are aware of benefits and help available, both from statutory and voluntary bodies.

Despite the many and diverse problems faced by the person who has had a stroke, there is frequently light at the end of the tunnel. Given adequate psychological support and the benefits of an integrated rehabilitation programme, many stroke patients develop a fulfilled, if profoundly changed, lifestyle. The outlook, both in terms of medical management and rehabilitation, is now a much more positive one. It is hoped that this book will make a useful contribution to this process by considering the theoretical and practical issues involved in both preventing stroke and in helping the stroke patient regain optimal independence.

Shorter stays in hospital, limitations on the hospital car service and restrictions on ambulance facilities in Great Britain, means that patients are not always receiving the long-term rehabilitation they need to restore optimum functioning. Given adequate resourcing and good team leadership, the concept of community care is a sound one; but the realities of the situation are sometimes in sharp contrast to the stated aims.

The shortage of places in specialist units and the difficulties which many patients face in obtaining adequate treatment is particularly frustrating at a stage where we can be increasingly optimistic about the effects of well-integrated and intensive programmes of rehabilitation. There is little doubt that therapy approaches have improved as a result of research, and this process has been facilitated by the move towards university training in the paramedical professions and greater demands for accountability. A small but increasing number of therapists now have research appointments which can lead to greater understanding of the efficacy of specific techniques.

Research can benefit the client in two ways: first, by helping us to understand the nature of the disability and, secondly, by specific efficacy studies into different treatment methods. With increasing emphasis on accountability and cost-effectiveness within the United Kingdom National Health Service, and virtually all health care systems internationally, it has become even more important to make sure that what professionals are doing is effective.

Research into the prevention and medical management of stroke now has an increasingly high profile, and we can look forward to a stage where advances in medical science will lead to the prevention of an increasing number of strokes. Similar advances in the field of biomechanics could lead to improved restoration of function in the hemiplegic patient. The application of computer technology has already enhanced the lives of severely disabled individuals including many with communication disorders.

Practical collaboration

MJ at the age of 47 suffered a sub-arachnoid haemorrhage which was subsequently aspirated at a major London hospital. When he returned to his local hospital he was singularly unresponsive toward his family and the ward staff and would stare quizzically at anyone who approached him but would say nothing. Concerned by this lack of response, the speech and language therapist decided to observe interactions with nursing staff, the physiotherapist and the occupational therapist. MJ responded more appropriately to the concrete, tangible demands of the others; but verbal or gestural approaches, whether from the family or professionals, were generally ignored.

Some weeks later, when assessed on the Boston Naming Test, the first breakthrough occurred when he looked at a line drawing of a bed and said 'posh bed'. For another week he said nothing more and would sit patiently looking at series of pictures with apparently minimal interest. His wife and teenage family found his behaviour bewildering and upsetting. MJ had always been known for his bizarre sense of humour, and they sometimes feared that he was still playing games with them.

His next material breakthrough came a month later when he suddenly read aloud a caption below a picture of a harbour in Scotland. He had occasionally uttered a single word when we were examining pictures, but this rarely bore any perceptible relation to the subject. There had been one or two instances when he would say a word which after much investigation appeared to have some relevance. MJ had a background in computing and, prior to his CVA, ran his own firm selling computers and networks. Both the speech and language therapist (SLT) and the occupational therapist (OT) were interested in exploring how far he had retained the knowledge and skills upon which his career had been based. His principal hobbies had been golf and cooking, particularly French cuisine.

Despite his restricted language output, he was able to express his disgust at being placed in front of a machine which he regarded as an antique. At the time an elderly BBC computer was the only machine which either the OT or the SLT had in their departments. Initially he displayed little apparent idea of how to operate the computer and scant familiarity with the keyboard, but both features began to show signs of improvement.

He was referred to a rehabilitation unit at a specialist hospital where he had intensive physiotherapy, occupational therapy and speech and language therapy. When he returned he showed marked improvement in all features of communication and mobility, but it was becoming obvious that he would be unlikely to return to his former work. His frustration made resettlement at home difficult but with the support of his family he was able to achieve a remarkable level of stability. Assessment by the clinical psychologist played a vital part in determining his suitability for an intensive rehabilitation programme and in monitoring his subsequent progress.

His computing skills continued to improve, and he was able to gain some

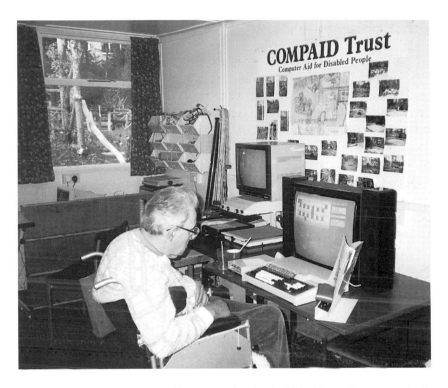

Fig. 1.1 A computer can facilitate writing even when the individual is unable to use a keyboard. Scanning phrases, word lists or the alphabet can be controlled by means of a single switch. With appropriate software, depending on the level of recovery, the individual can either communicate with speech output or in writing.

benefit from INTACT (*see* Appendix) and began to use a word processing program to write basic letters. Reduction of drive and initiative, associated with frontal lobe damage, initially restricted the recovery which he had been able to make; but he continues to attend a small high-level Action for Dysphasic Adults group and COMPAID (Computer Aid for Speech Impaired and Disabled People) where he continues to make progress in language skills and general confidence. He has started a part-time job, which gives him further focus and stimulation.

Collaboration in the earliest stages of recovery

The general practitioner, hospital medical and nursing staff are the initial group who may be involved in the care of the person immediately following a stroke. If swallowing difficulties are observed or suspected, the speech and language therapist is called in to assess and advise. The physiotherapist is usually also called in at this early stage and is principally involved with respiratory problems and mobility.

Dysphagia assessment

The collaborative nature of stroke care is exemplified in the process of assessment of dysphagia. The initial medical examination can give rise to concern that the patient has an absent gag reflex. From the nursing point of view it is not the gag reflex which is the pre-eminent problem but the individual's reflexive protection of his airway when swallowing fluids. Dysphagia occurs when the control mechanism for swallowing has been affected by the occlusion of arterial supply to the brain stem. Some patients show little or no sign of swallowing difficulties, others have problems which last for only a few days, whilst the remainder exhibit longer term or even permanent dysphagia. The latter situation tends to be related to successive bilateral cerebral infarctions affecting the motor areas.

It can be either the medical team or the nursing staff (see Fig. 1.2) who seek the involvement of the SLT. This usually occurs soon after admission to the ward; but if there is a log jam of patients because of a shortage of beds, it can even occur in the accident and emergency department. The initial step is to determine what has been observed by nursing staff in attempting to administer medication, fluids or food. In many cases the next stage is an assessment by the SLT which is often observed by the nurse involved with the patient. The patient's primary nurse is frequently involved in positioning the patient prior to the assessment.

The patient's response is discussed and recorded and recommendations are

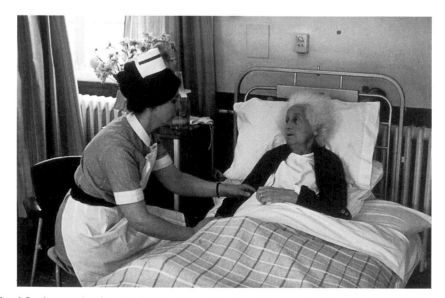

Fig. 1.2 A nurse is often the first member of the team to encounter the patient's difficulties with speech and swallowing.

made as to the viscosity of fluids which are likely to be safe, the need for insertion of a nasogastric tube or the desirability of performing a percutaneous endoscopic gastrotomy (PEG). This relatively simple surgical procedure allows the patient with poorly functioning swallowing mechanism to receive nutrition directly into the stomach. It is easily reversible and has made a considerable contribution to the care of individuals with severe long-term swallowing difficulties. The dietician is usually closely involved in such discussions and closely monitors fluid and semi-solid intake. In long standing cases such as Parkinsonian patients or those with Pseudo-bulbar palsy, who are admitted to the hospital for a period of acute care, family members or care staff can give valuable input to the team.

Some speech and language therapists, devoted to the intellectual challenges of working with the dysphasic adult, regard participation in the assessment of swallowing function as inappropriate especially when it tends to dominate the case load to the exclusion of linguistic rehabilitation. Others who find such work fascinating and fulfilling tend to defend their new territory. Few are, however, able to follow Logemann's (1995) dictum that bedside assessment should always be validated by video-fluoroscopy. She regards training the dysphagic patient to swallow effectively as more appropriate than solely identifying aspiration.

Few hospitals in the UK are able or willing to provide easy access to video-fluoroscopy. In many contexts such an examination would involve moving a very sick patient at best to another part of the same hospital or even some distance to another centre. In many instances the individual who has recently survived a stroke will not be able to cooperate in a video-fluoroscopic examination because it entails a high degree of compliance in both timing of the swallow and the general posture of the subject.

It is often difficult enough to perform a far less exacting bedside assessment, but the vast majority of cases are cooperative in spite of, in some cases, serious language difficulties and in others the possibility of confusion or deep depression because of the recent loss of function. One faces the ever-present risk that the lack of a protective response to the intake of fluid could mask a suppressed cough reflex. Preliminary discussion with nursing colleagues can usually help to determine the patient's main difficulties and provide valuable pointers towards assessment and management.

Where serious doubts arise about the efficiency of an individual's swallowing, it is essential that a video-fluoroscopic examination is arranged. Both radiologists and radiographers are closely involved with the patient who may be unable to understand instructions and comply successfully with the demands made for timing the intake of the barium solution and the optimal posture required for filming. Even in the most positive setting with skilled and understanding staff, the experience can be most distressing for the patient and result in equivocal findings. The relationship of trust and familiarity which has been set up on the ward between the patient and the speech and language therapist can help overcome the difficulties encountered in the video-fluoroscopy suite. Interpretation of the videofilm is usually a joint exercise, and a good working relationship between the radiologist and the SLT is of paramount importance. Each has much to learn from the other.

The dietician may prove to be the driving force in securing referral to the SLT and in particular re-referral after a prolonged period of nasogastric feeding. When the question of performing a PEG procedure is raised, the dietician plays a vital part in the decision making process.

Some physicians, as well as some SLTs, have questioned the role of the speech and language therapist in dysphagia assessment. One of the strongest positive arguments is that the assessor needs to be as sure as possible that the patient has understood and agreed to take fluid by mouth. In most cases explanation precedes the assessment, and the individual clearly assents to the procedure. Where the patient is confused or unable to understand the explanation offered, it is vital that the task is undertaken by someone experienced and skilled in coping with the language disordered individual and able to distinguish between confusion and communication disorder. Many speech and language therapists are now involved in training nursing colleagues to take over aspects of dysphagia assessment, but there have been recent calls for the establishment of a specific dysphagia therapist (Carrau *et al.*, 1998; Murray, 1998).

Dyspraxia assessment

The problem of dyspraxia also serves to illustrate a vital area of collaboration. Dyspraxia is one of the most puzzling and least well understood aftereffects of a stroke, even though it was clearly described over a century ago. The affected person shows no sign of paralysis in the speech mechanism or in a limb, understands the request made by the physician, nurse, physiotherapist or family member but appears totally unable to comply.

The speech and language therapist and the occupational therapist encounter more instances of dyspraxic behaviour because they undertake the assessment and rehabilitation of skilled behaviour. In recent years clinical psychologists have also become involved. Dyspraxia can affect any programmed pattern of movement including gesture and all aspects of spoken and written language (Square-Storer, 1989).

NT was a university administrator and an accomplished amateur musician prior to his CVA. His stroke left him with a right hemiplegia, a high level of understanding of language but a persisting inability to produce anything but a few unintelligible recurrent utterances and very restricted writing skills. He was totally incapable of playing an instrument which he had taught for years.

In the first twelve months following his stroke he made only limited progress in speech or other skills but began to regain his capacity to use a computer for specific exercises. He has been assessed for a portable communication aid with input from the OT, the SLT and his family, and it is hoped that he will begin to achieve greater levels of communication.

Collaboration with the family

One definite advantage of the current emphasis on dysphagia assessment is the opportunity to work with dysphasic individuals and their families from the very beginning of their difficulties. All too often in the past referral has been delayed because of a tendency to wait and see how the aftereffects of the stroke are manifested. Physiotherapy is typically introduced at an early stage because of the respiratory and mobility problems associated with stroke. Referral to the speech and language therapist can arise where the nurse or physiotherapist observes difficulties in comprehension of instructions or problems in expressive language.

A prime advantage of such early referral is the opportunity afforded to support both the patient and his family at a very distressing time. The family have a chance to ask questions and to observe interaction between their family member and an individual skilled in communicating with people with language disturbance. This can prove highly reassuring and influence all aspects of care. Reduction in the anxiety and distress shown by the family has a positive effect on the patient. The opportunity for relatives to meet others who have had strokes lays the foundation for more realistic aims with regard to the rate and extent of recovery which can be anticipated.

Some families spontaneously provide an ideal environment for the recovery of the member who has suffered a stroke. Others with appropriate guidance can learn to adapt to the individual's psychological and physical needs, but some will offer little comfort or support in spite of considerable input from professionals. The previous dynamics of the relationship between partners or within the wider family are crucial. Whitehead (1992) discusses the need for support groups for the relatives of dysphasic adults and describes some aspects of the work of the City Dysphasic Group. She cites Buck (1968) who describes stroke as a 'family illness'.

Family dynamics

Prior to her stroke AP was the dominant partner in both the home and the family business. She was originally left handed and following a right CVA survived with limited speech, severely restricted reading and writing and a left hemiplegia. All the humiliation and bullying which she had meted out to her husband in the past was now returned 'with interest' and added significantly to her feelings of loss and difficulties in adaptation. She had very great determination (she was a survivor of a concentration camp) and was spurred on to win back control of the business. Despite constant denial of progress she succeeded in regaining control of her speech, her family and the company.

JD was a careers advisor who worked in a major town but lived in a small rural community. She made a steady recovery of spoken language over a period of twelve months following a subarachnoid haemorrhage, but her written language recovered more slowly. She realized at an early stage that she would be unable to return to her former career, but the support from her husband and a network of

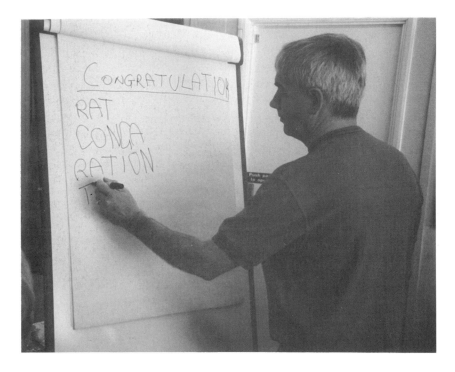

Fig. 1.3 Regaining writing skills is a major step towards building confidence.

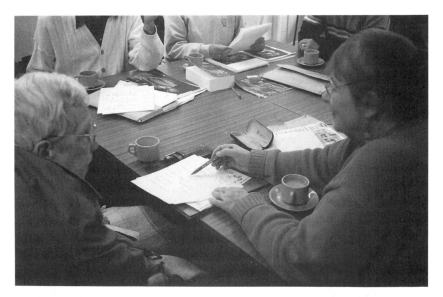

Fig. 1.4 A competitive element can be effective if members of a group are reasonably matched for communicative ability.

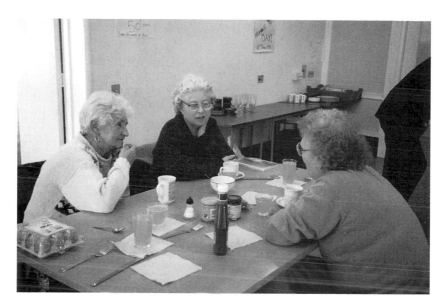

Fig. 1.5 Stroke groups and clubs facilitate communication because all the members have experience and understanding of the speaker's difficulties.

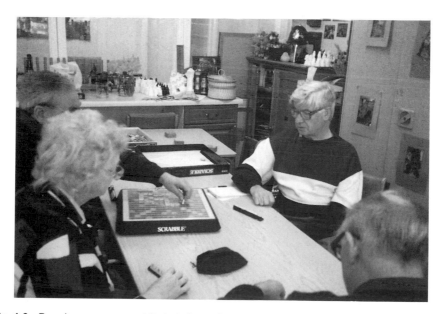

Fig. 1.6 Board games can contribute to improving motor control as well as communication skills.

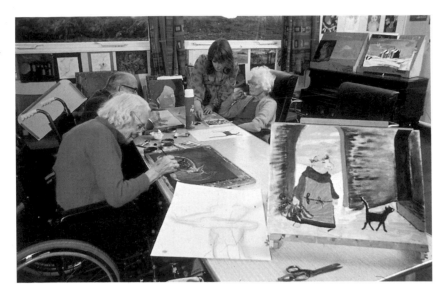

Fig. 1.7   Referral to an art therapist can provide opportunities for self-expression for an individual who is intensely frustrated by his or her communication difficulties.

friends in her village coupled with regular speech and language therapy resulted in a slow but marked improvement in both reading and writing. Her confidence in using spoken language has grown considerably, and she is now seeking ways in which she can use her former skills and abilities in the support of others who have experienced strokes. Even for the best adjusted family, there is much to learn, and the task of coping with the emotional difficulties alone would tax the most experienced professional who has the favourable advantage of relatively limited exposure to the problems.

The generic therapist

For some years there has been considerable discussion about the concept of a generic therapist who will deal with all aspects of rehabilitation. This idea has, not surprisingly, met with little enthusiasm from physiotherapists, occupational and speech and language therapists, but has the backing of some physicians and perhaps a larger number of administrators.

In view of the expertise and knowledge required to carry out all three therapies, it is difficult to see how any one person could fill all roles effectively. One can appreciate the principle behind the proposal. In the first place, the patient would have to cope with only one professional who would be cognizant of all aspects of his disabilities. The involvement of a single therapist would certainly overcome the problems of coordinating service delivery.

If the generic therapist is seen as a cost-cutting exercise, then it would seem to be on less solid ground. The generic therapist, having to manage all aspects of rehabilitation, would inevitably have a much smaller case load. There are already serious limitations on the time available for a given patient from each of these specialities. One can only assume that the concept of a generic therapist has been put forward by those who do not possess a complete understanding of what is involved in the work of each member of the rehabilitation team.

There is, of course, a measure of overlap in the aims and methods employed in all three therapies, but each member of the team has a unique role to play. This does emphasize, however, the importance of a coordinated team approach in stroke rehabilitation. The frustration encountered in being forced to restrict specific work in any of these fields, when the therapist is aware that concentration on a particular area could significantly benefit the patient, would lead to a major loss of job satisfaction and personal fulfilment, which would adversely affect morale. An alternative approach that has been carried out successfully in some centres involves the appointment of rehabilitation assistants who work with the patient under the direction of the appropriate therapist or combination of therapists. The rehabilitation assistants attend case conferences and are closely involved in the process of target setting and monitoring of progress.

Case conferences

Lubbock (1983), in her comprehensive account of interdisciplinary care for the stroke patient, states that 'the case conference is the hub round which members of the team work', but she also warns that 'it can become a tedious waste of time rather than something which increases efficiency'. The exchange of ideas and observations is a key factor in the organization of a rehabilitation programme, but the sessions need to be effectively chaired. It is essential that the views of all members of the team receive appropriate attention.

To pay mere lip-service to collaboration denies both the patient and the family their rights to a full and comprehensive service following a stroke. It is now more fully realized that the individual who has suffered the stroke is the most important member of the team. Participation in rehabilitation is never a passive role, but the individual may need considerable encouragement and support to achieve even the most basic steps and to realize the importance of his/her own contribution.

References

Buck, R. (1968) *Dysphasia: Professional Guidance for Family and Patient.* Prentice Hall, Englewood Cliffs, NJ.

Carrau, R.L. & Murray, T. (1998) *Comprehensive Management of Swallowing Disorders.* Singular Publishing, San Diego, Ca.

Logemann, J.A. (1995) Dysphagia: evaluation and treatment. *Folia Phoniatrica* **47**, 140–64.

Lubbock, G. (1983) *Stroke Care – An Interdisciplinary Approach*, pp. 16–9. Faber and Faber, London.

Murray, J. (1998) *Manual of Dysphagia Assessment in Adults.* Singular Publishing, San Diego, Ca.

Whitehead, S. (1992) Support Groups for the Relatives of Aphasic Adults. In *Group Encounters in Speech and Language Therapy* (M. Fawcus, ed.), pp. 89–100. Far Publications, Leicester.

Chapter 2

Medical Aspects of Stroke

Marion Hildick-Smith

Introduction

The World Health Organization (WHO) has defined stroke as a condition with 'rapidly developing clinical signs of focal loss of cerebral function, with symptoms lasting more than 24 hours or leading to death, with no apparent cause other than that of vascular origin.'

Stroke is a major killer and the cause of much disability, the management of stroke illness accounts for about 5% of NHS hospital costs. In the past it was an area of medicine that was neglected as dull and unrewarding, and it is only in the last two or three decades that this attitude has changed. There is now a great deal of research into the mechanisms of stroke damage, and the fields of prevention and rehabilitation are receiving attention, together with that of acute stroke care.

Epidemiology

Past studies of stroke incidence were bedevilled by inaccurate diagnosis, but as imaging techniques such as computerized tomography (CT) become more widely available, this will happen less often. Most epidemiological studies now use the WHO definition of stroke and attempt to include all identified cases whether seen at home or in hospital and whether elderly or not.

For example, the occurrence of stroke, including transient ischaemic attacks, has been under study in a general population sample of over 5000 men and women, followed over the last 34 years in the Framingham study (Kannel *et al.*, 1970). This prospective study gives the incidence of stroke in the 65–94 age group as 200 per 100 000 per year. This result is similar to those obtained by using pooled multinational data.

Under the age of 45 stroke is uncommon, although subarachnoid haemorrhage does occur in younger as well as older people. After the age of 45 the incidence of stroke doubles every decade (Kannel *et al.*, 1970 and 1981). About two-thirds of all strokes occur in people over the age of 70 years, and the average age of onset of stroke is 75 years. There is no adequate explanation of this great increase in stroke with advancing years. When allowance is made for the fact that women live longer than men, the sex incidence of strokes is equal.

Stroke is the largest killer in the UK and the USA after heart disease and cancer. In the United Kingdom middle class people are less likely than working class people to die from cerebrovascular disease, while in the United States, stroke is less prevalent among whites than among non-whites (Pickle *et al.*, 1997). Worldwide, the country with the greatest stroke mortality is Japan. Over the last 15 years, many Western countries have seen a progressive fall in deaths from stroke (Shahar *et al.*, 1995), though this decline may be slowing down (Gillum *et al.*, 1997). The variation in incidence of stroke in different countries has been decreasing (Sudlow *et al.*, 1997). No satisfactory explanation for the racial differences has been found, though dietary factors may play a part, as eating fresh fruit and vegetables may help to prevent stroke (Key *et al.*, 1996). In Britain, for example, the areas of lowest consumption of fruit and vegetables (the north and west) have higher stroke mortality than the southeast.

Strokes which resolve completely within 24 hours, called transient ischaemic attacks (TIAs), may not all be reported, so that their incidence is more difficult to determine than that of full strokes. An average incidence each year of TIAs of 31 per 100 000 population was reported in Rochester, Minnesota, over a 14-year period. The incidence rose steeply with age, and about a third of those with TIAs developed a full stroke in the next five years especially in the first six months (Cartlidge *et al.*, 1977).

Hypertension is the main risk factor for stroke, but other factors of importance include cardiac conditions such as left ventricular hypertrophy, or atrial fibrillation, and diabetes. Recently doubt has been cast (Jousilahti *et al.*, 1997) on whether a positive family history is an independent risk factor for stroke, low birth weight may be a risk factor for men (Martyn *et al.*, 1996). For middle-aged people, factors such as a raised haematocrit or fibrinogen level may be important. Environmental factors of significance include cigarette smoking which increases the risk of stroke by 3.5, and exposure to cold (The Eurowinter Group, 1997). Either non-drinking or heavy drinking is a risk factor, but moderate drinkers may benefit because of their increase in high density lipoprotein-cholesterol. Exercise has not shown direct benefit but may help because it leads to weight reduction and promotes a healthier lifestyle.

Survival clearly depends on the type of stroke and on the age of the stroke victim. In the early weeks of the illness, about half of all stroke patients will die. Those who survive this period may succumb to further strokes (Hankey *et al.*, 1997) or heart attacks in the first year, and few stroke survivors live for ten years after the onset of their illness.

Stroke is the biggest cause of serious physical disability. Of more than 100 000 first strokes each year in the UK, 60% will be dead or dependent in activities of daily living 6 months later (Sandercock & Lindley, 1993). There are about 130 000 stroke survivors living in the community in the UK, of which about three-quarters are severely handicapped (Cifu & Lorish, 1994), predominantly with hemiplegia, cardiovascular disease, speech or mental problems. However, the picture is more hopeful for those who show useful recovery and can return home – a third of these return to normal activities and one in ten has no remaining deficit. We do not know why stroke patients recover, and the needs of patients at home after stroke are only now being systematically studied.

The decline in the incidence of stroke and of deaths from this condition over the last few decades shows that stroke is neither the inevitable consequence of ageing nor the inescapable result of genetic constitution.

Aetiology

It used to be thought that stroke always occurred because of vascular disease within the brain. It is only in the last three decades that the role of the extra-cranial arteries and the heart in stroke has been clarified. We have also become humbler about our ability clinically to distinguish between the three main types of strokes – cerebral thrombosis, cerebral haemorrhage and cerebral embolus. We are readier to use the general term 'stroke' until imaging studies enable us to make the specific diagnosis.

Roughly 85% of acute strokes are due to the blockage of a cerebral artery by a solid clot of blood (cerebral thrombosis), which leads to cerebral infarction (Hyman, 1992). Atheroma may build up at sites on intracranial and extracranial arteries where there is turbulence or mechanical stress and lead to blockage. Alternatively, the source of the blockage may be an embolus (a travelling clot) which has recently lodged, for example, at the site where the common carotid artery divides in the neck. These emboli usually arise from the heart valves or walls. Blockage in a large vessel leads to a wedge-shaped cortical infarct, visible on CT scan, whereas when deep penetrating cerebral arteries are involved, small deep lacunar-shaped infarcts are seen near the internal capsule and thalamus. (These previously unsuspected lesions explain some puzzling presentations of stroke.)

The remaining 15% of acute strokes are due to cerebral haemorrhage from small intracerebral arteries which have developed microaneurysms, usually as a result of chronic hypertension (Hyman, 1992). The commonest site of a massive haematoma is within the basal ganglia leading to downward displacement of the brain, when death may arise, commonly in 2–7 days, from pressure on the brain stem.

We know that the brain has no reserves of the sugar and oxygen it needs to maintain its metabolic requirements. A cerebral infarct is an area of brain in which the blood flow has fallen below the level required to maintain the tissues in a viable state. Early on, the infarct is swollen and softened but difficult to delineate. Over 3–4 days the lesion becomes well-defined and the swelling is greatest. Older infarcts have a clear outer edge, and the centre of the infarct may dissolve and cavitate over the next three months.

A gradient of blood flow exists after complete blockage of a blood vessel. The central zone has no bloodflow but the periphery or penumbra, which is ischaemic and swollen, may not be irreversibly damaged. It may show normal or increased blood flow and may have potential for early intervention treatments. The mechanism of ischaemic damage may be via free radical species, because the normal superoxide dismutase which scavenges these species is impaired and the free radicals become available as toxins. They may also be generated during reperfusion when oxygen again becomes available. Such damage may be prevented if neuroprotective agents can be developed and deployed early after a stroke.

The joins (anastomoses) which occur normally in brain blood vessels at the base of the brain (in the circle of Willis) or between large vessels, like the external carotid and internal carotid, make it possible for blood to reach the periphery by backflow along an anastomosis, thus also limiting the damaged area.

Of cerebral infarcts, 75% occur in the territory of the middle cerebral artery, 15% in the vertebrobasilar artery territory and 10% in the border zones between two major arteries (so-called 'watershed' infarcts) (Hyman, 1992). Blockage of the middle cerebral artery, or of the internal carotid artery, gives rise to damage in frontal and parietal lobes of the brain leading to hemiplegia (paralysis of arm and leg on the opposite side of the blockage), sensory loss, language disturbance, perceptual problems and hemianopia. If the branch to the internal capsule is blocked, there will be motor hemiplegia only.

Damage to the anterior cerebral artery is a rarer cause of stroke and causes paralysis of the leg but not the arm, and may lead to urinary incontinence due to damage to the frontal lobe which controls voluntary micturition. Infarction of the posterior cerebral artery leads to altered consciousness, brain stem loss, including cranial nerve palsies, hemiplegia, blindness and cerebellar symptoms. Sometimes the damage may be bilateral due to blockage of the basilar artery. Abbreviations which are increasingly used are those of total or partial anterior circulation infarct (TACI and PACI) and posterior circulation infarct (POCI) and lacunar circulation infarct (LACI).

'Watershed' infarcts are an important cause of strokes in elderly people, the junction of the middle and anterior cerebral arteries being most vulnerable. The cause may be a period of progressive hypotension (low blood pressure) leading to poor perfusion to the 'last fields of irrigation' of the relevant artery. Alternatively, showers of small emboli may arise (e.g. from the carotid bifurcation).

'Lacunes' are small irregular softenings up to 1.5cm in diameter, occurring often in the basal grey nuclei. They may be silent or, if repeated, may lead to a 'L'etat lacunaire', a progressive stepwise deterioration with dementia, pseudobulbar palsy and shuffling gait. The cause of this syndrome is not clear, but it may be due to micro-atheroma or to replacement of the cell walls of the tiny vessels with fatty hyaline material.

In Binswanger's syndrome, there are multiple lacunes in the basal nuclei and also in the white matter of the brain which shows areas of demyelination (Zhang & Olsson, 1997). Affected patients usually show hypertension, and there is usually atheroma of basal cerebral arteries and of small cortical vessels. This syndrome is more readily diagnosed since the advent of CT scanning, as the diffuse low-density lesions in the white matter can be readily seen.

Cerebral haemorrhage (accounting for 15% of strokes) is frequently a complication of high blood pressure, though an increasing number of haemorrhagic strokes in elderly demented people are secondary to amyloid changes in small vessels. Subarachnoid haemorrhage occurs when a small berry aneurysm on the circle of Willis bursts, leading to bleeding into the subarachnoid space and sometimes also into the cerebral tissue. The 'berry' aneurysms are now thought to be acquired, not congenital, and unruptured aneurysms are described in 2% of all routine post-mortems. Overall, the commonest site of massive cerebral haemorrhage is within the basal ganglia, in the area supplied by the perforating branches of the middle cerebral artery. The cause is not clear, though lipohyaline changes in small vessels may predispose to tiny leaks, causing a false aneurysm which may later rupture.

Clinical features

Since the diagnosis of stroke (WHO) is purely clinical, a thorough clinical assessment is necessary if management is to be effective. The clinical features of stroke depend on the site and extent of brain damage, and no two patients are identical. The first difficulty facing the doctor is to decide whether the patient has had a stroke or not. For example, the patient may have had a *grand mal* fit followed by Todd's paralysis (postepileptic weakness), giving rise to a hemiplegia which resolves completely in up to 48 hours. Alternatively, there may be a history of an old stroke, making the new neurological signs difficult to distinguish. A more dramatic illness, such as a cardiac infarct or serious fracture may overshadow the signs of accompanying stroke so that the diagnosis is missed. A history of head injury with impaired or fluctuating level of consciousness out of proportion to the signs of 'stroke' may indicate a subdural haematoma. Neoplasm elsewhere (such as in the breast or the bronchus) may not have been diagnosed; and the semi-acute history of stroke may be due to a brain metastasis. Acute hypotension (due to a gastrointestinal bleed, silent myocardial infarct, dehydration or drugs) may mimic a stroke, as may hypoglycaemia (from long-acting antidiabetic medication). Non-specific presentations of stroke in the elderly include sudden confusion, incontinence of urine or falls, or there may be a misleading history of alcohol excess.

Often it is necessary to examine a patient several times over the course of days, to confirm changes in signs and performance and to judge whether there was an initial stroke or not. Even with careful observation the clinician may miss the diagnosis of stroke in up to 33% of cases or may diagnose stroke when it is not present in up to 22% of patients, when compared with diagnosis at post-mortem, or by CT and/or magnetic resonance imaging (MRI) (Ebrahim, 1992).

The clinical differentiation between cerebral haemorrhage and cerebral infarct is not very accurate. Signs suggestive of cerebral haemorrhage include initial loss of consciousness, headache, vomiting, neck stiffness and blood in the cerebro-spinal fluid. These two latter signs occur only if blood leaks into the subarachnoid space, so a small haemorrhage may be difficult to differentiate from a thrombosis. CT scanning performed within two weeks of onset of stroke is the most widely available investigation that can reliably detect primary intracerebral haemor-rhage (Hankey & Warlow, 1994), and there is now pressure for such scanning to be done very quickly after a stroke. This issue is becoming more important as antithrombotic treatment should now be considered for a patient with cerebral thrombosis, but could be disastrous for one with cerebral haemorrhage.

Motor loss from stroke can result from a lesion in the brain stem, up to the level where the motor fibres cross to the opposite side in the pons, or from tracts in the internal capsule up to the motor cortex in the frontal region. The most obvious clinical feature of most strokes is the weakness which affects one side of the body (hemiplegia). The arm is nearly always involved, but leg weakness is less prominent or sometimes absent; and this distribution is characteristic of a middle-cerebral artery lesion. Weakness affecting predominantly the leg is rare and indicates an anterior cerebral artery blockage. Severe loss of muscle function is associated with an increased mortality rate. Muscle tone control is complex and many different tone patterns are found with damage to different parts of the brain. These lesions interfere in different ways with the underlying tone of the muscles and the facilitatory and inhibitory influences on them via the reflex areas. Classically, the hemiplegia will be accompanied (after initial flaccidity) by increased tone in the flexors of the arm and extensors of the leg. (One aim of nursing and therapy positioning and treatment is to prevent the development of this abnormal spasticity.) Some patients continue with hypotonia, which has a very poor prognosis for mobility, especially if accompanied by perceptual or cognitive deficit.

Motor function depends on adequate feedback, so interference with sensation from the limbs is usually accompanied by some motor dysfunction. Sensory messages (touch, pin prick, deep pressure or proprioception) pass from the sensory nerve endings up to the opposite side of the brain along sensory nerves via the thalamus. A lesion at this site can give rise to sensory disturbance accompanied by distressing 'thalamic pain' so that the patient has to avoid touching anything with the affected side, as this is likely to set off the pain. Higher interpretation of sensations takes place in the primary sensory cortex (just pos-terior to the motor cortex) where the leg area is represented at the top and there is disproportionate representation lower down of the hands and fingers, feet and lips. Damage at this level (cortical sensory loss) is tested by blindfolding the patient and giving him an object to feel in his affected hand. He may be able to move the object in his hand but cannot tell what it is – whether sharp or blunt, hot or cold, heavy or light. Unless such a patient can compensate by looking, for example, at his clothes, he will have great difficulty in dressing himself.

Further analysis of sensory information occurs in the secondary (association) cortex in the parietal lobe. Damage to this area may lead the patient to be totally unaware of the affected side (hemisomatognosia) and he may be unable to use that side unless continually reminded of it, though it is not paralysed. These sensory problems are a grave barrier to recovery. The patient may deny any problem (anosognosia) and insist that he can dress, and walk, though he fails to do so and has no perception of what is required.

Visual problems may result from stroke. Normally the impulses from the left side of visual space are picked up by the right side of each eye and travel back to the right occipital cortex. Hence damage to the nerves before they reach the cortex results in blindness to the left side of space. The patient will be aware of his problem and will try to avoid bumping into things by turning his head and eyes to compensate for the deficit. If the stroke damage is in the occipital cortex, the patient may not only be blind for half of space but also unaware that there is a deficit. This visual neglect may include leaving half of his meal, or drawing only half of a clock, as he has no awareness that he should try to overcome his deficit. Visual memory may be lost so that the patient 'forgets' where the sleeve is when he looks at the collar – this obviously makes dressing very difficult. Trying to stimulate the affected side by putting food, drink or photographs there will fail if the patient has no awareness of deficit. Similarly, it is better for the nurse and relatives to approach from the 'good' side – otherwise they will not be recognized.

Communication is one of the most important higher functions of the brain and disturbance of speech can be one of the most isolating aspects of stroke. If the speech reception area (Wernicke's area) in the parietotemporal area is damaged, interpretation becomes impossible, as does feedback, so the patient talks fluent gibberish and cannot take in what is said (executive and receptive dysphasia). The motor component of speech is mainly organized in the frontal lobe (Broca's area). Damage to this area gives rise to difficulty in finding the correct word for an object or person (nominal dysphasia) and sometimes to total inability to speak (expressive aphasia). Other speech difficulties in stroke include: a. dyspraxia – inability to control the muscles of tongue and lips, though they may work automatically on occasions; b. dysarthria – in which speech is slurred because face and tongue movements are weakened; and c. dysphonia – when the laryngeal muscles are weak and sounds cannot be produced. The latter two are usually related to stroke lesions in the brainstem. (A more detailed explanation of speech disorders is given in Chapter 7.)

Emotional control is a function of the brain, and we normally keep tight control over our emotional reactions. Loss of this controlling function due to a stroke lesion leads to emotional lability (being moved easily to tears or laughter). It can also lead to distressing emotional incontinence, when the patient bursts into uncontrollable weeping at the slightest provocation, while being fully aware of this problem. The syndrome is particularly common where bilateral strokes have occurred and is part of the picture of pseudobulbar palsy. Accompanying signs may include weak and spastic arms and legs, problems with swallowing and a hoarse voice.

Brain stem lesions can result in a severe stroke because even a small lesion can cause a lot of damage. In addition to signs of hemiplegia, there may be loss of sitting balance (ataxia) and dizziness, paralysis of ocular muscles, dysarthria and dysphagia (problems of swallowing). Often the patient is unconscious with abnormal cyclical breathing (Cheyne-Stokes) and the prognosis then is very poor. Occasionally the above symptoms may be due to a large cerebral haematoma or haemorrhage distorting the anatomy of the brain and causing pressure on the brain stem.

Problems of swallowing were in the past thought to occur only where both hemispheres were involved over the years by stroke damage. However, it is now clear that about one-third of patients with a single hemiplegia have dysphagia in the early weeks after stroke (Gordon *et al.*, 1987). It depends on whether the swallowing control centre is in the R or L hemisphere. With recovery of swallowing (which occurs in 90% of patients by three months) control switches to the other side of the brain (Hamdy *et al.*, 1997).

Some patients have an abrupt onset of suspected stroke, progressing rapidly to coma, but have no focal neurological signs. This can occur with catastrophic intracranial haemorrhage, but another surgically treatable alternative (in suitable patients) is a cerebellar stroke which will be visible on CT scan.

Shoulder pain on the affected side is found frequently in stroke patients. Flaccidity of muscles around the shoulder leads to poor support, with subluxation of the humerus which stretches the shoulder capsule and rotator cuff. Further damage to the shoulder can be done by poor lifting – pulling the patient up by the affected arm, or using the axilla as a leverage point. Correct lifting techniques performed by *all* who help the patient can be effective in reducing this further distress to the patient.

Depression occurring soon after a stroke is a common part of the grief reaction, as the patient mourns his past healthy and active role in life. Depression many months after stroke may be due to failure to adapt to the stroke or may be due to a specific effect of localized brain damage. Although symptoms of depression may be difficult to clarify (e.g. appetite and bowel problems may be due to inactivity), surveys have suggested that significant depression occurs in up to a third of stroke patients and is poorly recognized (Robinson & Price, 1982). Tricyclic antidepressants may be of limited value because of their serious side-effects in the elderly (confusion, constipation, etc.); but alternative antidepressants and/or supportive psychotherapy are being studied, as they might be of value, as might attendance at a stroke club.

Cerebrovascular disease is responsible for one-fifth of the dementias, though the mechanism is unclear (Pasquier & Leys, 1997). The term multi-infarct dementia may be inappropriate, as infarcts are not always present. The predominantly male and hypertensive patients have usually had at least one stroke and have shown a stepwise deterioration in their mental state. (This is in contradistinction to Alzheimer's dementia where the deterioration is smooth and gradual, though the two forms of dementia can coexist.)

Deep small lesions in the region of the internal capsule can cause pure motor stroke without any cortical impairment, one of the lacunar syndromes. These syndromes are probably under-diagnosed in the elderly, and information about their natural history is lacking.

Transient ischaemic attacks can show any of the varied signs and symptoms of a completed stroke, but there is complete resolution within 24 hours. The question arises whether the symptom is caused by vascular disease or by migraine or epilepsy. The latter would come on more slowly and might progress to unconsciousness which is rare in TIA. The distinction between TIA and a Todd's paralysis following epilepsy can, however, be difficult to make. The importance of making the diagnosis of TIA lies in the fact that 30% of affected patients go on to have a full stroke in the next few months. These strokes may be prevented by relevant medical or surgical treatment.

Examination of the patient

Many of the signs which are relied on to diagnose a stroke and estimate its severity are imprecise and may be interpreted differently by different examiners. The signs usually recorded (muscle power and tone, reflexes and plantar responses) are not necessarily the most important ones for diagnosis, management or prognosis. The patient may tire during a prolonged examination, and score poorly on mental testing or perceptual tests. To combat these problems many units are now standardizing the questions asked on a printed sheet, though it may not be feasible or desirable to ask them all at once.

During admission, the crucial decisions are whether the patient has had a stroke and whether other treatable causes of neurological symptoms and signs have been excluded. This necessitates finding out the patient's symptoms and their speed of onset, confirmed if possible by a spouse or carer. (If the onset has been over days, then subdural haematoma, cerebral tumour or abscess are possible alternatives.) A list of the patient's medication is needed. Treatment, for example, with a long-acting hypoglycaemic drug for diabetes may suggest that the neurological signs will probably disappear when the blood sugar is brought back to normal. Signs suggestive of meningitis should be sought, so that antibiotic treatment can be given. It is helpful to have details (from patient or carer) of the patient's capabilities (physical and mental) and the degree of help he or she has needed prior to the present episode so that the degree of recovery can be estimated. It is also necessary to know whether the patient can swallow or not, and whether steps will need to be taken to prevent pressure sores.

Examination of the nervous system will reveal few or many signs according to the site and extent of the lesion which has caused the stroke. The patient's level of consciousness should be assessed and monitored if there is cause for concern. Signs localizing the lesion to one side of the body suggest a hemiplegia or hemi-sensory loss. Bilateral signs may indicate a brain stem lesion, or a severe cerebral lesion distorting the anatomy within the skull and pressing down on the brain stem. Alternatively there may have been a previous hemiplegia on the other side from the present one.

If there is motor loss it is helpful to assess the patient's function such as 'can he or she shrug shoulders or cock back their wrist' (these actions may have to be demonstrated first). These functional losses can be monitored and will give some idea of progress and prognosis.

Multiple pathology is common in old people, so full examination of an elderly person with a stroke will be needed. For example, the patient's pulse may show atrial fibrillation and his blood pressure may be high. The doctor will need to assess whether these findings are consequent upon the stroke, unrelated to the stroke or important in the causation of the stroke. This is often a difficult issue to decide. Atrial fibrillation (AF) is present in 8% of women, and in 13% of men over 80 and is associated with a five-fold increase in the risk of stroke (Wolf *et al.*, 1978) so anticoagulants for uncomplicated AF should be considered (Singer, 1996). Left ventricular hypertrophy is not easy to confirm clinically – but if present, it would suggest that any hypertension is of some duration.

Chest examination may show signs of previous problems which will increase the likelihood of, for example, aspiration pneumonia following the stroke. The breathing may show the Cheyne-Stokes pattern, which has a poor prognosis.

General examination may show evidence of a neglected neoplastic lesion, e.g. in breast, chest or abdomen, and the neurological signs may be due to a metastasis. The legs may show varicose veins, or the leg arteries may show poor blood supply, suggesting widespread cardiovascular disease. The neck may show a bruit over the carotid artery. During the examination the doctor may be able to assess the patient's response to the stroke, including mental ability, mood and morale, all of which will be crucial in determining the like-lihood and degree of recovery.

Investigation of the stroke patient

Investigations of stroke in the elderly may need to be more numerous, partly because of the non-specific presentation of the disease in some cases, and partly because clear histories are often difficult to obtain at the time of admission. In addition, many treatable non-vascular causes of stroke are more common in older patients. It is advisable to check the blood count and erythrocyte sedi-mentation rate (ESR), the blood sugar and electrolytes, the VDRL (a test for syphilis), chest X-ray and electrocardiogram. The first two may yield information suggestive of anaemia or polycythemia or cranial arteritis. Increased levels of fibrinogen or cholesterol may also be relevant in younger stroke patients or in those with ischaemic heart disease. The blood sugar may be low due to long-acting hypoglycaemic drugs, may be slightly raised due to the 'stress' of the stroke, or may be very high in diabetic coma. The electrolytes may show dehydration or the low sodium and potassium of sick elderly people. 'Cardiac' enzymes may be suggestive of recent cardiac infarct. The VDRL may give evidence of syphilis, while the chest X-ray may show a neoplasm or severe infection. The ECG may show a silent infarct (leading to a period of hypotension or to a mural thrombus and embolus). It may confirm an arrhythmia such as atrial fibrillation. Evidence of left ventricular hypertrophy on the ECG suggests that hypertension has been lengthy. Echocardiography may be indicated to clarify abnormal findings on the chest X-ray or the ECG, or where positive blood cultures suggest endocarditis. It may also be useful in a younger stroke patient where no cause for the stroke can be found.

Special investigations in appropriate patients would include ultrasound duplex testing of the carotid arteries for well elderly people who are suspected of having TIAs. Carotid angiography may reveal that the corresponding carotid artery has a blockage of greater than 70%, in which case carotid endarterectomy would be considered. For those with less than 29% blockage, medical management with aspirin is advised.

Computerized tomography has gradually established its place as a diagnostic tool in stroke, and within the first 10 days is positive in 100% of those with cerebral haemorrhage and in 80% of those with cerebral infarcts. A CT scan can differentiate stroke from subdural haematoma, cerebral tumour or abscess and can demonstrate the stroke lesion in the cerebellum in some puzzling cases. Differentiating cerebral haemorrhage from cerebral thrombosis will become increasingly important as early treatment for cerebral thrombosis with anti-platelet or anticoagulant or thrombolytic drugs is considered. For example, if the CT scan is reasonably normal, thrombolytic drugs can be given to reperfuse the arteries and reduce the damage, though there is always a small risk of haemorrhage (Furlan & Kanoti, 1997).

Magnetic resonance imaging (MRI) has a higher sensitivity for early cerebral infarcts than CT scanning. It can show up smaller lesions and is better at revealing those in the posterior fossa. It is helpful in prognosis, as patients showing infarct volume of greater than 100 cm^3 are very likely to die or be severely dependent. With special new techniques diffusion MRI can show the lesion in 4 hours and this technique may be a selective marker for necrotic tissue damage. However, it is not widely available.

Clinical features predictive of poor outcome include age, previous stroke, urinary incontinence, altered consciousness at onset, etc. (Kwakkel *et al.*, 1996). Research is being done on blood tests which may help to predict outcome, including hyperglycaemia, serum S100, glutamate and glycine (Castillo *et al.*, 1997).

Perfusion imaging, a different technique, can show the larger area at risk of infarction. The difference between perfusion MRI and diffusion MRI is the ischaemic penumbra, which might be potentially rescuable in the future. Coupled with MR angiography, the precise site of the arterial occlusion can be identified. This could be of great importance in the future if the indications for thrombolysis are clarified and the results of treatment could be followed. MR angiography can also identify 'berry' aneurysms as small as 10 mm in diameter and can outline carotid stenosis. A further new technique, functional MRI, has the potential for identifying brain tissue with preserved function. It can follow the apparent reorganisation of cerebral motor pathways following injury and would be useful to evaluate rehabilitation techniques. MRI is less widely available than CT and most of the newest techniques are confined to a few research centres.

References

Cartlidge, N.E.F., Whisnant, J.P. & Elveback, L.R. (1977) Carotid and vertebrobasilar transient cerebral ischaemic attacks; a community study, Rochester, Minnesota. *Mayo Clin. Proc.* **52**, 117–20.

Castillo, J. *et al.* (1977) Progression of ischaemic stroke and excitotoxic aminoacids. *Lancet* **349**, 79–83.

Cifu, D.X. & Lorish, T.R. (1994) Stroke rehabilitation; 5 stroke outcome. *Archives of Physical Medicine and Rehabilitation* **75**(S), 56–60.

Ebrahim, S. (1992) Diagnosis. In *Oxford Textbook of Geriatric Medicine* (J.G. Evans and T.F. Williams, eds), pp. 313–18. Oxford University Press, Oxford.

Furlan, A.J. & Kanoti, G. (1997) When is thrombolysis justified in patients with acute ischaemic stroke? *Stroke* **28**, 214–18.

Gillum, R.F. *et al.* (1997) The end of the long-term decline in stroke mortality in the United States. *Stroke* **28**, 1527–9.

Gordon, C., Langton Hewer, R. & Wade, D.T. (1987) Dysphagia in acute stroke. *BMJ* **295**, 411–14.

Hamdy, S. *et al.* (1997) Explaining oropharyngeal dysphagia after unilateral hemispheric stroke. *Lancet* **350**, 686–92.

Hankey, G.J. & Warlow, C.P. (1991) The role of imaging in the management of cerebral and ocular ischaemia. *Neuro-radiology* **33**, 381–90.

Hankey, G. *et al.* (1997) Stroke recurrence over 5 years after first-ever stroke in Perth, Western Australia. *Cerebrovascular Diseases* 7 suppl. **4**, 75.

Hyman, N.M. (1992) Pathology of stroke. In *Oxford Textbook of Geriatric Medicine* (J.G. Evans & T.F. Williams, eds), pp. 297–303. Oxford University Press, Oxford.

Jousilahti, P. *et al.* (1997) Parental history of cardiovascular disease and risk of stroke; a prospective follow-up of 14,371 middle-aged men and women in Finland. *Stroke* **28**, 1361–6.

Kannel, W.B. *et al.* (1970) Epidemiologic assessment of the role of blood pressure in stroke: the Framingham Study. *Journal of the American Medical Association* **214**, 301–10.

Kannel, W.B. *et al.* (1981) Systolic blood pressure, arterial rigidity and risk of stroke: the Framingham Study. *Journal of the American Medical Association* **245**, 1442–5.

Key, T.D. *et al.* (1996) Dietary habits and mortality in 11,000 vegetarians and health-conscious people: results of a 17-year follow-up. *BMJ* **313**, 775–9.

Kwakkel, G., Wagenaar, R.C. *et al.* (1997) Predicting disability in stroke – a critical review of the literature. *Age and Ageing* **25**, 479–89.

Martyn, C.N., Barker, D.J. & Osmond, C. (1996) Mother's pelvic size, foetal growth and death from stroke and coronary heart disease in men. *Lancet* **348**, 1264–8.

Pasquier, F. & Leys, D. (1997) Why are stroke patients prone to develop dementia? *J. Neurol.* **244**, 135–142.

Pickle, L. *et al.* (1997) Geographic variation in stroke mortality in blacks and whites in the United States. *Stroke* **28**, 1639–47.

Robinson, R.G. & Price, T.R. (1982) Post-stroke depressive disorders: a follow-up study of 103 patients. *Stroke* **13**, 635–41.

Sandercock, P.A. & Lindley, R.I. (1993) Management of acute stroke. *Prescribers' Journal* **33**, 196–205.

Shahar, E., McGovern, P.G., Spraflea, J.M., Pankow, J.S., Doliszny, K.M., Leupker, P.V. & Blackburn, H. (1995) Improved survival of stroke patients during the 1980s. The Minnesota Stroke Survey. *Stroke* **26**, 1–6.

Singer, D.E. (1996) Anticoagulation for atrial fibrillation: epidemiology informing a difficult clinical decision. *Proceedings of the Association of American Physicians* **108**, 29–36.

Sudlow, C.L.M. & Warlow, C.P. (1997) The International Stroke Incidence Collaboration. Comparable studies of the incidence of stroke and its pathological types. *Stroke* **28**, 491–9.

The Eurowinter Group (1997) Cold exposure and winter mortality from ischaemic heart disease, cerebrovascular disease, respiratory disease, and all causes in warm and cold regions of Europe. *Lancet* **349**, 1341–6

Wolf, P.A., Dawber, T.R., Thomas, H.E. & Kannell, W.B. (1978) Epidemiologic assessment of chronic atrial fibrillation and risk of stroke: the Framingham Study. *Neurology* **28**, 973–7.

Zhang, W.W. & Olsson, Y. (1997) The angiopathy of subcortical encephalopathy (Binswanger's Disease). *Acta. Neuropathica* **93**, 219–224.

Chapter 3
Medical Management of Stroke
Marion Hildick-Smith

Acute stroke

The question of whether patients should be admitted to hospital is not clearcut, and currently one-third of stroke patients are managed at home. The general practitioner (who will see three or four stroke patients a year) will make this decision, usually based on the patient's home circumstances (availability of carer, etc.) and on the adequacy of the community nursing and support services available. The GP may also take into account the age of the patient and the severity of the stroke, as many families will wish their relatives to die at home. Admission to hospital to clarify the diagnosis and facilitate early treatment and rehabilitation is rarely suggested by GPs, though hospital consultants, especially those with designated stroke units, regard these aspects as very important. In the management of acute stroke, the history, examination and investigation of the patient are crucial, as detailed throughout this book.

In the past the place of specific treatment has not been clear nor has there been evidence of benefit from the use of haemodilution, naftidrofuryl, glycerol, mannitol or high-dose corticosteroids in acute strokes (Bath, 1995). However, two major trials of antiplatelet and antithrombotic therapy have now been reported. A randomized study of 20 000 patients (Chinese Acute Stroke Trial, CAST, 1997) showed that treatment with 160mg aspirin per day within 48 hours of ischaemic stroke (confirmed in 87% of cases by CT scan) was beneficial and should be continued. It led to a reduction both in mortality and in recurrent strokes in the first weeks. The equally large randomized and controlled International Stroke Trial (IST, 1997) showed similar benefit from 300mg aspirin a day. However, heparin at over 5000 IU twice daily gave rise to a significant increase in cerebral haemorrhage.

These two very large studies show that aspirin should be given within 48 hours of ischaemic stroke. In the longer term, aspirin should be continued to prevent another stroke. Men and women of all ages, hypertensive or not, can benefit – in fact, the higher the risk factors, the greater the benefit. The dose of aspirin is still strongly debated (Hart & Harrison, 1996). Most doctors start with 150–300mg daily reducing the dose progressively to one or even half of a 75mg tablet daily if dyspepsia occurs.

The place of thrombolytic therapy is still being clarified and depends on the balance between risk and benefit for each individual. In a recent review of published trials, the risk of cerebral haemorrhage averaged 10.3%, and there was a 40% increase in the odds of death among fibrinolysis-treated patients (Furlan & Kanoti, 1997). There is a possibility that some subgroups might benefit. Selection factors such as early CT changes, severe stroke or age over 77 years might exclude those least likely to benefit; but it is still not possible to predict response to treatment in individual patients. Further carefully designed trials are needed to clarify this issue.

The National Institute of Neurological Diseases and Strokes (NINDS) rtPA Stroke Group has suggested that a system should be set up to treat hyperacute stroke with rtPA (recombinant tissue plasminogen activator) within three hours of stroke (NINDS, 1997).

Low levels of serum ionised magnesium are found in patients early after stroke and are claimed to cause spasm in the cerebral vessels (Altura *et al*, 1997), so the place of intravenous magnesium is currently being investigated in the Images trial. These trials confirm the need for early admission and CT scanning to identify patients who can benefit from aspirin and any other new treatments. An Oxford study (Salisbury *et al.*, 1998) of 153 patients admitted to hospital with acute stroke in 1997 showed that patients who went straight to hospital by ambulance suffered least delay in assessment (2 hours, 12 minutes from onset) compared with those who called a GP. The study concluded that if acute therapies for stroke became available, general practitioners should be the primary targets for an educational initiative. Certainly a patient with a mild stroke should not be advised to wait and see whether it is a TIA.

Swallowing difficulties occur in up to half of acute stroke patients and are often missed by medical and nursing staff. Speech therapists have developed an important role here as part of the 'swallowing team', which may also include a doctor, a nurse and a dictician. The decision whether to start artificial feeding in the first 24 to 48 hours needs careful consideration in each case, though it is helpful to have a locally agreed policy. In some patients evidently dying of stroke, whose relatives do not want medical intervention, it may be agreed that such treatment is inappropriate. A similar situation may arise when the patient has previously been incapacitated by other strokes, by dementia, or by serious heart or chest problems or neoplasia. Over 20% of all stroke patients die within a month. Frequent discussion with nurses and relatives about the prognosis and about aspects of management must take place and the issue must be sensitively handled.

Patients who have previously had a good quality of life, and where stroke is less disastrous, will benefit from intravenous or nasogastric feeding or by insertion of a PEG (percutaneous endoscopic gastrostomy) tube. This will improve their nutrition and help to avoid dehydration, pressure sores or other complications of stroke. In a small randomized prospective study of 30 patients with acute stroke (Norton *et al.*, 1996) PEG feeding emerged as better than nasogastric (NG) feeding in decreasing mortality, improving nutrition and increasing likelihood of discharge from hospital. The researchers recommend that PEG treatment should be the method of choice in appropriate stroke patients. A further study is also currently researching whether dietary supplements are associated with better outcome after stroke.

Half of all hemiplegic patients will develop a deep vein thrombosis (DVT). The International Stroke Trial found that subcutaneous heparin in doses of up to 5000 IU per day would be helpful in prevention. Physical methods of DVT prevention, such as graded compression stockings, can be used to reduce the incidence by 60–70% without any risk of cerebral haemorrhage.

For incontinence due to stroke, an external penile catheter may be needed in men and an indwelling catheter in women. These should be avoided if possible, as they lead to urinary infection. As soon as the patient is conscious, the catheter can be taken out and incontinence managed with regular toileting and the use of pads. Bowel function must be watched and care taken to avoid constipation or faecal impaction.

Frequent turning is required to prevent pressure sores, and a physiotherapist will advise nurses on positioning the patient in bed and in a chair and on attempts to balance and stand. A physio will also demonstrate how patients can be moved without pulling on a paralysed arm and shoulder. Educated help from nurses is crucial in every aspect of patient care – the amount of help to be given with feeding and conversation and assistance to the patient in setting goals (see Fig. 1.1).

Hypertension is the single most important risk factor for stroke, and the reduction of blood pressure reduces the risk of stroke. It is doubtful whether reduction of blood pressure immediately after a stroke is beneficial. Blood pressure tends to fall spontaneously in the first days after stroke, and any decision to give hypotensive drugs should take account of the fact that cerebral blood flow (CBF) is altered after stroke. Cerebral autoregulation is lost for up to several weeks, so CBF may depend on the blood pressure. Rapid decrease in blood pressure in the first few days may, therefore, make the situation worse. Current advice is to watch the blood pressure for three or four days and if necessary to start hypotensive drugs carefully after this period. Patients who have had strokes or TIAs are at greater risk of serious recurrence than asymptomatic people with high blood pressure in the general population. So treating the high blood pressure in the high-risk population will bring greater absolute benefit.

Over 10% of patients with strokes have fits that may require anticonvulsant treatment in the acute stage after stroke. In a substantial group these drugs may be withdrawn after a few weeks without recurrence. However, in the remainder, the fits may persist (perhaps arising from an area of scarring where the infarct occurred) and treatment needs to continue.

All stroke patients who smoke should be advised to stop. Those who stop, at any age, will soon benefit from the increase in their life expectancy. There is no evidence that alcohol intake affects the risk of stroke in the old or that obesity justifies changing the diet, though increasing fruit and vegetable intake may be beneficial. The fact that agitation and depression are common in stroke must be remembered, so that not too many unwelcome pieces of advice are given at a time of great stress. One of the benefits of getting patients up and dressed and of helping with mobility, as soon as this is advisable, is that the patient's morale and self-image are improved by these manoeuvres. One piece of good advice for couples is that they can resume their normal sex life, as it is not dangerous to do so after stroke so long as high blood pressure has been treated.

The indications for carotid endarterectomy in acute stroke and TIA are becoming clearer, and perhaps GPs should be encouraged to refer more elderly people for duplex scanning. The patient must be fit for the operation and must have made a good functional recovery from a stroke in that part of the brain supplied by the internal carotid artery.

The blockage in the ipsilateral (symptomatic) carotid artery must be greater than 70% on carotid duplex scanning (ECSTCG, 1991), which is a non-invasive investigation. Many neuro-surgeons will say that the results of carotid angiography (which carries a 1–2% risk of stroke) must be available as a prerequisite for surgery (which itself carries a 4–5% risk of stroke). Where the carotid blockage is <30%, medical management is advised, as it is for 30–70% (ECSTCG, 1996). Where carotid blockage is asymptomatic, endarterectomy is not at present indicated (ECSTCG, 1995). Randomized controlled trials of carotid angioplasty and also of inserting stents into the carotid are currently being undertaken, to see if they provide useful alternatives for selected patients.

Rehabilitation

Rehabilitation from stroke starts from the day of admission in the positive and hopeful attitude which staff communicate to the patients and relatives. It works via the multidisciplinary team's complex assessment of the patient's physical, mental, social and spiritual needs. This includes assessment of disability (e.g. need of help to dress) and handicap (with regard to the patient's social roles in employment and leisure activities). There is an element of planning (analysing the problems and setting achievable goals) which should be undertaken with the patient's active cooperation. Rehabilitation includes intervention to reduce the disability and handicap and checking on the effects of the intervention.

The overall level of physical disability must be assessed, and there are numerous scales which can be used including the Motricity Index and the Rivermead Motor Assessment. However, the Barthel index of Activities of Daily Living (ADL) is widely used clinically and includes aspects of bowel and bladder function, grooming and toilet use, feeding, transfer from bed to chair, mobility, dressing, ability to climb stairs and to bath independently (Wade & Collins, 1988). Tests of mental function include the Glasgow Coma Scale (an important indicator of prognosis) and the 10-question Mental Status Questionnaire (for orientation and short-term memory) (Hodkinson, 1972). The Frenchay Aphasia

Screening Test (FAST) is a short test for detecting and quantifying aphasia (Enderby *et al.*, 1986).

A limited number of the above tests (and of other relevant ones) are used at any time, as stroke patients tire quickly, especially if elderly. Based on the information available from the patient, from relatives or carers, and from the multidisciplinary team meetings, a plan is made for achievable goals in order to enlist the patient's cooperation and improve morale. As progress is made, further goals can be set. One important goal can be planning the patient's discharge and smooth transfer to the community services. This may entail knowledge of the patient's current ability in activities of daily living (ADL) and safety; the motivation and mood of the patient and of any carer; the suitability of his house; the provision of aids such as walking frame or wheelchair; the need for cooking or household tasks to be arranged; liaison with community services and with day care or relief care; and the need for follow-up, including day-hospital and home therapy.

The natural history of stroke must be taken into account. About 30% of patients will die in the first 3 months, most of those dying from the stroke itself during the first 3 weeks. As mentioned in a previous chapter, patients most likely to die are those with the most severe strokes, as shown by loss of consciousness, gaze palsies, complete paralysis, incontinence and swallowing difficulties. Those who are still incontinent 2–3 days after suffering a stroke are more likely to die or to need long-term institutional care. Over the first week about 20% of patients show deterioration, presumably due to further cerebral infarction, while others will show rapid fluctuation or improvement. Once the clinical state has settled, a 2–3 week period of rapid recovery occurs, followed by slower but continuing improvement over 3 months. Those who show no voluntary handgrip after 3 weeks are unlikely to regain useful arm function, and the same applies to speech in aphasic patients. The chance of much improvement overall after 6 months is low.

Relatives will need a lot of information from doctors and nurses about stroke, and the leaflets published by the Stroke Association make a very helpful and readable contribution. The latest two of these, published in 1998, give advice on rehabilitation and information for carers. Stroke Family Support Workers are greatly valued by stroke families, although research has failed to identify more than marginal effects (Dennis *et al.*, 1997). Similar results apply to specialist nurse support in the community (Forster & Young, 1996), so further investigation is needed to discover what sort of person is needed to give support. Relatives need to know that long-term 'rest' is not beneficial and that early mobilization improves the patient's morale and helps to prevent abnormal tone, deep vein thrombosis, etc.

The rehabilitation efforts of a multidisciplinary team are something of a 'black-box' and it is difficult to research which aspects of rehabilitation are helping. To help with this a Stroke-Association-funded Therapy Research Unit opened in 1997 in Salford. Even in well-staffed units patients will receive treatment for only 3.5 hours during the patient's 'working' day. Some research suggests that it is the early timing of the therapist's input which is important rather than total quantity

(Smith *et al.*, 1981). 'Intensive' treatment, however, has given even better results in some studies. Skilled observation is needed to separate out those patients who are depressed at 3 months and need antidepressants from those who cry because of 'emotional incontinence', as previously described. Counselling for both patient and family can often be of benefit, especially when they are coming to terms with the fact that active treatment is not likely to lead to further improvement.

Long-term, about half of stroke survivors will be left with some physical disability and about 5–10% will need long-term institutional care. Local authorities are now responsible for the care of many of these patients, as are numerous private and voluntary homes, as hospital long-term care beds have virtually disappeared. Early assessment after the stroke will enable the physician to identify those who need help and ensure that they receive whatever is available, in order to reduce dependency.

Little allowance is made in public places and on public transport for people with physical disability, and so they suffer considerable handicap. It is important to many who recover from a stroke to continue driving, and wherever possible (legally, financially and in terms of safety) this should be made a goal of treatment. Loss of driving capability is strongly connected with depression. There are welcome signs that cars adapted to the needs of elderly drivers are being designed. Putting the patient and/or carer in touch with day-centres and support groups such as stroke clubs may be of help. They may be able to advise about state benefits which can be claimed, and will organize social activities and provide information and support.

Overall, the available evidence from 19 trials shows that organized forms of rehabilitation (stroke teams, stroke wards and stroke units) are better than routine hospital care (Stroke Unit Triallists' Collaboration, 1997). Specialist units reduce early mortality for up to a year and improve the functional outcome in survivors. A recent Danish study (Jorgensen *et al.*, 1995) showed that stroke units also reduced hospital length of stay as well as costs.

The forms of stroke care vary within countries and between countries. Some stroke units, for example, take acute stroke patients, while the majority concentrate on rehabilitation. What they all have in common is an enthusiasm for treating stroke patients, and many of their policies could be disseminated more widely by stroke teams within hospital or at home. The King's Fund Consensus Conference (1988) on the treatment of stroke recommended that an integrated stroke service should be built up in every locality, to give better treatment and information to stroke patients and their carers.

Prevention of stroke

As brain tissue, once lost because of stroke, cannot be replaced, there is a limit to what rehabilitation can achieve. The best way forward is to learn how to prevent strokes in the first place.

As already stated, strokes predominantly occur in older people: 70% of strokes happen to people over 65, and older victims are more likely to die from a stroke. The fact that the likelihood of suffering a stroke increases with age suggests that there may also be an accumulating environmental factor involved. There is considerable variation in the incidence of stroke between different countries, and this may possibly be due to different dietary habits or, for example, different water hardness. Another piece of evidence for an environmental factor is that stroke incidence and mortality has decreased in many Western countries over the last four decades. The reason for this decline is not yet clear.

Elderly people particularly at risk from stroke include those with high blood pressure, diabetes, peripheral vascular disease, previous TIA or stroke, atrial fibrillation, and clinical or ECG evidence of coronary heart disease. The dominant risk factor for stroke in elderly people is high blood pressure. Stroke is seven times as common in people with high blood pressure; and the higher the blood pressure, the greater the risk of stroke. It seems clear, therefore, that high blood pressure should be treated, and there may be greater benefit from treating older patients. However, the decision to treat hypertension in elderly people is not straight-forward. High blood pressure is common in elderly people, and it has been taught that blood pressure increases with age: the diastolic pressure peaks in middle age and then declines, whereas the systolic pressure peaks at age 70 and over – so the elderly often show isolated systolic hypertension (Evans, 1987). This was present in 18% of men and 30% of women over 75 and was also predictive of stroke.

Some elderly people, on the other hand, show a decline in blood pressure with age and may need to come off their previous hypotensive drugs. Measurement of blood pressure in the elderly is not easy, and they may show 'pseudohypotension' due to decreased compliance of the artery walls. Reduction of systolic high blood pressure can reduce the risk of stroke in selected elderly people kept under careful surveillance (SHEP, 1991). Benefit has been shown in patients aged up to 80, but larger studies are needed for patients over 80 with careful balancing of side-effects against potential benefits. Even a small reduction in blood pressure can bring benefit, e.g. reducing the diastolic pressure by 5mm Hg (Macmahon & Rodgers, 1996) can reduce risk by one-third, so the readings do not necessarily need to be brought down to 'normal' levels.

Although the combination of a thiazide diuretic (hydrochlorothiazide 25mgm) with triamterene (50mgm) was used in the European Working Party on High Blood Pressure in the Elderly (Amery *et al.*, 1985) with good results, these drugs would no longer be a first choice for hypertension in the elderly. A calcium channel blocker such as adenosepine, which has fewer side-effects, would be preferred.

Beta-blocker treatment is often contra-indicated in elderly people who have bronchospasm or peripheral vascular disease because of the feeling of fatigue which it causes in full doses. However, in low dosage, e.g. 25mgm atenolol, it can be effective and troublefree. If beta-blockers cause problems or are contra-indicated, an ACE inhibitor can be used.

Atrial fibrillation is a risk factor for stroke leading to a fivefold increase in incidence, especially if there is also valvular and ischaemic heart disease. Some elderly people who go in and out of atrial fibrillation (AF) may be at particular risk. Meta-analysis of six major clinical trials (Morley *et al.*, 1996) showed the four independent clinical features that increased the risk of stroke in patients with AF. These were hypertension, increased age, previous TIA, and diabetes mellitus. Without anticoagulant therapy, patients with AF and any of these risk factors had a 4% annual risk of stroke. Patients with AF and congestive cardiac failure or coronary artery disease have three times the risk of stroke as do those without concomitant features. Patients with AF but no other risk factors seemed to have little concomitant risk of stroke. Overall these studies showed a 64% reduction in risk of stroke in patients treated with warfarin compared with a placebo. Attention was drawn to the increased risk of haemorrhagic complications in those over 75.

Another study in 1996 (Anon. Stroke prevention in AF 111, 1996) sought a safer alternative to fixed-dose warfarin in high-risk patients (those with AF and one other risk factor for stroke). More than 1000 patients were randomly allocated to one of two treatment regimens: fixed-dose low-intensity warfarin and aspirin, or adjusted-dose warfarin (aiming for an INR of 2 to 3). The trial was stopped after a year when those on adjusted-dose warfarin showed 6% less ischaemic or embolic strokes than those on fixed-dose combined therapy, while risks of major bleeding were similar in both treatment groups.

Those suffering transient ischaemic attacks (TIAs) are at higher risk of stroke especially during the first year after the TIA. Treatable causes of TIAs (giant-cell arteritis, embolism from the heart, etc.) need to be identified, and the degree of blockage of the carotid arteries studied by Doppler scanning. For appropriate patients who have stenosis of the carotid artery of more than 70%, an urgent operation to unblock the artery (endarterectomy) will reduce the risk of stroke. Aspirin also reduces the risk of further stroke, and lower doses such as 150mgm a day, are as effective as higher ones and give less risk of any side-effects.

Cigarette smoking is a risk factor for stroke in younger patients. Although the relative risk declines with age, it is still worthwhile to advise older people to stop smoking. Older people should avoid exposure to cold, as there are higher rates of stroke at times of high wind-chill. There is no convincing evidence that alcohol intake affects the risk of stroke in the old or that obesity or raised blood lipids justify dietary interference to change stroke risk. However, this situation may change as cohorts of middle-aged people live into old age, having been exposed to lower lipid levels than are current in developed countries. Eating more fruit and vegetables is beneficial. Snoring as a risk factor in stroke is currently being investigated and may be associated with increase in platelet aggregation in the early hours of the morning.

There is consensus now that treatment of hypertension and advice to stop smoking should be part of the treatment of all people at high risk of stroke or after stroke. Nevertheless, the application of this advice by GPs is variable around the country (Du, X. *et al.*, 1997) and training may be needed to emphasize the importance of prevention. By treating hypertension in middle age and in later life, by investigating patients with TIAs, and by instituting healthier lifestyles in middle age, further reduction in stroke incidence in old age may be possible in the future.

References

Altura, B.T. *et al.* (1997) Low levels of serum ionised magnesium are found in patients early after stroke which result in rapid elevation in cytosolic free calcium and spasm, in cerebral vascular muscle cells. *Neuroscience Letters* **230**, 37–40.

Amery, A. *et al.* (1985) Mortality and morbidity results from the European Working Party on high blood pressure in the elderly trial. *Lancet* **i**, 1349–54.

Anon (1996) Adjusted-dose warfarin versus low-intensity, fixed-dose warfarin plus aspirin for high-risk patients with atrial fibrillation. (Stroke Prevention in Atrial Fibrillation 111 randomised clinical trial.) *Lancet* **348**, 633–9.

Bath, P.M.W. (1995) Treating ischaemic stroke: still no effective drug treatment available. *BMJ* **311**, 139–40.

CAST (1997) Randomised placebo-controlled trial of early aspirin use in 20,000 patients with acute ischaemic stroke. *Lancet* **349**, 1641–9.

Dennis, M. *et al.* (1997) Evaluation of a stroke family care worker: results of a randomised controlled trial. *BMJ* **314**, 1071–7.

Du, X. *et al.* (1997) Case-control study of stroke and the quality of hypertension control in north-west England. *BMJ* **314**, 272–6.

(ECSTCG) European Carotid Surgery Triallists' Collaborative Group (1991) MRC European Carotid Surgery Trial: interim results for symptomatic patients with severe (70–99%) or with mild (0–29%) carotid stenosis. *Lancet* **337**, 1235–43.

ECSTCG (1995) Risk of stroke in the distribution of an asymptomatic carotid artery. *Lancet* **345**, 209–12.

ECSTCG (1996) Endarterectomy for moderate symptomatic carotid stenosis. Interim results from the European Carotid Surgery Trial. *Lancet* **347**, 1591–3.

Enderby, P.M. *et al.* (1986) The Frenchay Aphasia Screening Test: a short simple test for aphasia appropriate for non-specialists. *International Rehabilitation Medicine* **8**, 166–70.

Evans, J.G. (1987) Blood pressure in stroke in an elderly English population. *Journal of Epidemiology and Community Health* **41**, 275–82.

Forster, A. & Young, J. (1996) Specialist nurse support for patients in the community: a randomised controlled trial. *BMJ* **312**, 1642–6.

Furlan, A.J. & Kanoti, G. (1997) When is thrombolysis justified in patients with acute ischaemic stroke? *Stroke* **28**, 214–18.

Hart, R.G. & Harrison, M.G. (1996) Aspirin wars: The optimal dose of aspirin to prevent stroke. *Stroke* **27**, 585–7.

Hodkinson, H.M. (1972) Evaluation of a mental test score for assessment of mental impairment in the elderly. *Age and Ageing* **1**, 233–8.

(IST) The International Stroke Trial (1997) A randomised trial of aspirin, subcutaneous heparin, both or neither among 19,435 patients with acute ischaemic stroke. *Lancet* **349**, 1569–81.

Jorgenson, H.S., Nakayama, H., Raaschou, H.O., Larson, K., Hubble, P. & Alsen, T.S.O. (1995) The effect of a stroke unit: reductions in mortality, discharge rate to nursing home, length of hospital stay and cost. A community-based study. *Stroke* **26**, 1178–1182.

King's Fund Consensus Conference (1988) Treatment of stroke. *BMJ* **297**, 126–8.

Macmahon, S. & Rodgers, A. (1996) Primary and secondary prevention of stroke. *Clinical and Experimental Hypertension* **18**, 537–46.

Morley, Y. *et al.* (1996) Atrial fibrillation, anticoagulation and stroke. *American Journal of Cardiology* **77**, 38A–44A.

(NINDS) National Institute of Neurological Diseases and Stroke rt-PA Stroke Study Group (1997) A systems approach to immediate evaluation and management of hyperacute stroke. *Stroke* **28**, 1530–40.

Norton, B. *et al.* (1996) A randomised prospective comparison of percutaneous endoscopic gastrostomy and nasogastric tube feeding after acute dysphagic stroke. *BMJ* **312**, 13–16.

Salisbury, H.R., Banks, B.J. *et al.* (1998) Delay in presentation of patients with acute stroke to hospital in Oxford. *R. Jour. Med.* **91**, 635–40.

SHEP Co-operative Research Group (1991) Prevention of stroke by antihypertensive drug treatment in older persons with *isolated systolic* hypertension. Final results of Systolic Hypertension in the Elderly Program. *Journal of the American Heart Association* **265**, 2255–64.

Smith, D.S., Goldenberg, E. *et al.* (1981) Remedial therapy after stroke: a randomised controlled trial. *BMJ* **282**, 517–20.

Stroke Unit Triallists' Collaboration (1997) A collaborative systematic review of the randomised trials of organised in-patient (stroke unit) care after stroke. *BMJ* **314**, 1151–9.

Wade, D.T. & Collin, C. (1998) The Barthel Index: a standard measure of physical disability? *International Disability Studies* **10**, 64–7.

Chapter 4
Nursing the Patient Following a Stroke

Graham Boswell

Definitions of nursing are varied and focus upon different aspects such as the therapeutic interpersonal process in Peplau's model (1952) to the identification of need, appropriate intervention and evaluation of action identified by Wiedenbach (1964) (both cited in Chinn & Kramer, 1991). These reflect the different roles, practices and directions of nursing care within the multiple contexts that nursing operates. As no definition is comprehensive to all nursing practice, the care identified in this chapter will be that nursing is the assessment of patient/carer need and the management of available resources to meet that need.

Nursing as a process can be seen to follow a Gestalt principle in that the sum of the whole is greater than the sum of the parts, which consist of sociology, psychology, biology, physiology etc.; but the application of these knowledge bases to addressing the needs of an individual creates more than just the theories. A chapter on nursing people following a stroke can do no more than give nurses more knowledge or help organize their knowledge, so that they can make more informed decisions abut patient care. It can also provide colleagues in contiguous fields with insights into the decision-making processes and the principal issues involved in nursing patients after a stroke.

As can be seen by this book, the effective management of people following a stroke is not the prerogative of any particular healthcare profession but a combined approach from all. Nurses, especially within the hospital framework, possess a unique position within this multi-disciplinary approach. Due to the nature of their work, other therapists offer intensive therapy for the patient and guidance for other professionals; however, nurses have the opportunity to gain a greater insight into the patient, through greater contact whilst providing 24-hour care. They also have the opportunity to facilitate seamless care by ensuring continuity of practice as well as to mediate nursing concerns through their own and others' practice. However, for the care to be effective, the patient, their carers and all appropriate health professions must work together to achieve realistic goals.

The assessment of patient need and appropriate response relies upon understanding what is physically happening to the patient, the likely responses of the patient and their carers and the resources which can be brought to bear upon the situation. As such, the chapter will first briefly review the physical effects of a stroke upon the patient before exploring the potential nursing care needs of a patient. Accurate examination of a patient's nursing care need requires a systematic structure, a nursing model. The nursing requirements for most patients following a stroke are a process of rehabilitation. A nursing model that is focused towards a rehabilitation approach is that described by Orem (1985, cited in Aggleton & Chalmers, 1986). The model identifies eight universal healthcare needs that must be satisfied by an individual who is healthy. These are:

- sufficient intake of air
- prevention of danger to the self
- sufficient intake of water
- sufficient intake of food
- satisfactory eliminative functions
- activity balanced with rest
- time spent alone balanced with time spent with others
- being 'normal'

Following a stroke an adult may have difficulty fulfilling one or more of these activities, i.e. have a healthcare deficit that may result from (Aggleton & Chalmers, 1986):

- a lack of knowledge
- a lack of skill
- a lack of motivation
- past experience

The role of the nurse is therefore to accurately assess with the patient what healthcare deficits exist and then what interventions are appropriate to address these deficits. Interventions can be wholly compensatory (such as passive limb exercises), partly compensatory (such as walking with an unstable patient) and educative/supportive (teaching and motivating somebody to stand independently). Having identified the deficit and the appropriate response, the role of the nurse is to carry out that activity and to evaluate its effectiveness in collaboration with the patient. Reflection upon action enables the care to evolve to meet the patient's changing needs (Aggleton & Chalmers, 1986).

To review the nursing care of patients following a stroke, this chapter will first briefly review the effects of a stroke in order to put the potential nursing care in context. It will then follow the structure of the universal healthcare needs to systematically identify potential problems and nursing interventions. As in all nursing care, the ABC (airway, breathing & circulation) assume first priority until assessed as safe or compensated for. Other issues of care follow these essentials of life.

Effects of a stroke

An in-depth analysis of the causes and effects of a stroke are detailed in Chapter 2. However, for the planning of the nursing care a person will require following a stroke, a brief summary of the stroke process and its effects will provide a basis for the consequent nursing action.

Whether a stroke is caused by the obstruction of an artery or an intracerebral bleed, there is a wedge shaped disruption to the blood supply of the nerves after the point of insult. In the centre of the wedge the cells die around the time of the insult, but on the edges of the disruption the cells may be kept 'alive' by the collateral circulation. The autoregulation of blood supply within the brain will mean that as carbon dioxide levels rise in the interstitial spaces of the damaged area, then blood pressure will rise and collateral circulation will increase in an attempt to adequately supply this area. Disruption in the flow of nutrients and oxygen to and from cells will lead to the build-up of interstitial fluid, i.e. oedema, a swelling that acts as a space occupying lesion. These lesions put pressure on surrounding tissues, potentially disrupting their normal blood supply and increasing the number of cells at risk of death from ischaemia (Tortora & Anagnostakos, 1990 & Shepard & Fox, 1996).

From a nursing perspective the immediate management of a person's care after a stroke is aimed at supporting the nerve cells that are compromised but not yet dead and reducing the threat to the surrounding tissues, i.e. keeping the person alive and limiting the potential damage. In the longer term it is in ensuring that the person is able both to regain control of functions, controlled by areas of the brain that are impaired but not completely destroyed, and to adapt to any residual deficit.

Immediately following a stroke the person may suffer a loss of function, consciousness or their life. The immediate loss of function indicates which brain cells are at the heart of the ischaemic area and at most potential risk of permanent damage. Over the next three to four days as oedema and disruption to blood supply compromises the surrounding tissues, the impairment to the patient's function is liable to increase. The blood pressure is liable to rise but not necessarily in a problematic way. The level of anxiety felt by patients and relatives is liable to rise as the patient 'worsens'. As such, the patient gets worse before getting better, but the management of nursing care needs to accommodate these expected processes.

Sufficient intake of air

A stroke may affect the person's ability to swallow, their level of consciousness and their ability to maintain their own airway. As a sufficient intake of air is essential for life, it is vital that the patient's capacity to maintain a sufficient intake of air is assessed on admission and evaluated throughout their care. With an unconscious or semi-conscious patient, the use of the recovery position will help maintain their airway; and the deeply unconscious person may require the use of an airway or intubation. If there is any concern about the efficiency of respiration, then oxygen saturation can be monitored without discomfort to the patient and humidified oxygen therapy may be prescribed (Hickey, 1977).

Assessment of any swallowing difficulty requires assessment by the speech and language therapist. Interventions may require exercises or alterations to diet such as thickening fluids to make them easier to swallow. The greater viscosity slows down the transfer through the pharynx and reduces the risk of aspiration. If the swallow reflex is sufficiently impaired, then nasogastric or PEG feeding may be indicated.

Aspiration and period of lying static following a stroke may encourage the development of chest infections. Assessment by the physiotherapist, video-fluoroscopy, chest X-ray, a sputum sample sent for culture and sensitivity should identify the extent and the type of any problem. Treatment may consist of deep breathing exercises, chest physiotherapy, antibiotics, bronchodilators, sputum pots and tissues. The appropriate interventions depend upon an accurate assessment of the patient's needs.

Prevention of danger to the self

Observations

Management of the acute patient is based upon the appropriate assessment of need. Neurological observations using the Glasgow Coma Scale is the most widely used tool for the assessment of patients with altered levels of consciousness. However, its value in the assessment of stroke patients is limited except for those undergoing streptokinase therapy. The coma scale is a numerical value of consciousness constructed from a score of 1–4 for the patient's ability to open their eyes, 1–6 for the motor response and 1–5 for the verbal response. With a maximum score of 15 and a minimum score of 3, in the absence of extraneous circumstances, the lower the score, the greater the amount of disruption of cerebral activity (Frawley, 1990 and Hickey, 1997).

The pattern of a stroke, namely ischaemic damage, swelling, raised blood pressure and possible break up of 'clot' will result often in a deteriorating level of consciousness without the stroke worsening or extending. The coma scale is seen to be most effective when used every 15 minutes to a maximum of 30 minutes by a trained and experienced practitioner (Rowley & Fielding, 1991). Most importantly, however, it is only effective when a change in score will impact upon treatment. If this is not the case, then the observations may cause pain, distress, anxiety and disruption of sleep/rest in the patient, all of which can contribute to raising their intracranial pressure and inhibit recovery. However, for patients not undergoing streptokinase therapy, the coma scale can be effectively used to monitor a patient's condition as a daily assessment. This does not mean that observations (for most stroke patients) should not be carried out but that less intrusive ones (pulse, blood pressure and mean arterial pressure) may produce the important information.

In the 3–6 hours following a stroke the option of treating an occlusive stroke (caused by a clot) with streptokinase may be available. This reduces the size of the clot and the extent of the blood supply disruption to nerve cells, thereby improving the patient's prognosis. This is only available to patients who satisfy certain criteria but some attempts are being made to increase the number of patients to whom this is available (Hickey, 1997). For these patients, as for all stroke patients, the nursing care will focus upon the identification of a patient's nursing needs and the resolution of those needs. For this group it will be appropriate to monitor their neurological condition using the Glasgow coma scale for the first 24–48 hours and respond appropriately. Their nursing need will, as for all stroke patients, depend upon the extent and type of disruption caused by the stroke. As such, the chapter will focus upon post-stroke nursing needs, which may be applicable to all.

Hypertension

Different perceptions of the greatest threat to patients following a stroke will determine the response to treating hypertension. Both perceptions are valid and are grounded in the physiology of a stroke and its effect upon the person. Decisions to treat or not are determined by the cause of the stroke. In treating hypertension the focus is upon reducing the likelihood of a rebleed by reducing the pressure upon the clot and preventing vasogenic oedema (the osmotic movement of fluid into the interstitial spaces to balance the leaked plasma). This approach is appropriate in the management of the patient whose stroke is caused by haemorrhage. When not treating hypertension, the approach is seen as positive to the patient's outcome. This is due to the higher pressures being required to improve the collateral blood supply and to compensate for disruptions to the normal autoregulatory system. Limiting the amount of tissue receiving an inadequate perfusion reduces cytotoxic oedema, and is appropriate to the management of occlusive strokes (Shepard & Fox & Hickey, 1997).

Autoregulation maintains cerebral perfusion through a response to carbon dioxide levels and pressure within the cerebral arteries. A rise in the levels of carbon dioxide and hydrogen ions causes a dilation of local/cerebral arteries and a consequent increase in the amount of oxygenated blood reaching those tissues. A fall in the amount of carbon dioxide leads to a constriction of those blood vessels. A rise in the pressure within the artery leads to a dilation of that vessel, and a fall in pressure leads to a constriction of the vessel. The result is a flexible supply of blood able to meet the varying needs of cerebral tissues and the maintenance of sufficient pressure to maintain the perfusion of those tissues (Hickey, 1997).

In order for blood to enter the essentially 'closed box' of the skull and the brain, the blood pressure must be higher than the pressure of the skull's contents. Cerebral perfusion pressure is the blood pressure gradient required to perfuse the brain. It is the difference between the incoming arterial pressure and the opposing intracranial pressure, i.e. the following formula:

$$\text{Cerebral perfusion pressure} = \text{Mean arterial pressure (MAP)} - \text{Intracranial pressure}$$

In order to calculate this, it is first necessary to calculate the formula for the mean arterial pressure:

$$\text{MAP} = \frac{\text{systolic} - \text{diastolic}}{3} + \text{diastolic}$$

If someone's blood pressure was 150/90, this would mean that his/her MAP would be:

$$\frac{150 - 90}{3} + 90 - \frac{60}{3} + 90 = 110$$

Intracranial pressure can only be measured via an intracranial bolt, which is rarely used with stroke patients in the UK, and means that for most stroke patients the cerebral perfusion pressure cannot be measured. Normal MAP is between 60 and 150mm Hg, with hypertensive patients tending to the higher end of this range. A reduction of MAP by 16–25% will induce failure of the auto-regulatory mechanisms and result in hypoperfusion of the brain. A reduction of MAP by 50% will lead to cerebral ischaemia. As such, the measurement of blood pressure will give a good indication of the perfusion of the brain (Shepard & Fox, 1996; Hickey, 1997).

Pain

Pain in the acute phase of a stroke (1–2 weeks) is usually a severe headache due to meningeal irritation from blood and/or raised intracranial pressure (Hickey, 1997). The nursing intervention is to assess the extent and nature of the pain by verbal and non-verbal clues as well as tools such as pain charts. The nurses then ensure the physical comfort of the patient (positioning, pressure area etc.), minimize irritating stimuli such as noise, give analgesia as prescribed and needed, and monitor its effectiveness as well as ensuring that the patient understands what is happening and why, as knowledge can reduce the impact of pain (McCaffery, 1979).

Chronic pain is usually orthopaedic in nature and arises from the subluxation of joints, especially the shoulder from the weight of a flaccid arm. Prevention of this pain comes from passively exercising and supporting the limb. Analgesics will provide relief of this pain as may some complementary therapies. However, some chronic pain may result from lesions within the central nervous systems, especially associated with the thalamus. Relief from this pain is more effective with the use of either antidepressants or anticonvulsants and occasionally with the use of opiates (Segatore, 1995).

Rehabilitation

Andrews (1987) defines rehabilitation as 'the restoration of optimal levels of physical, psychological and social ability within the needs and desires of the individual and his/her family' (Tyson, 1995). The extent and range of dysfunction following a stroke is unique to the individual. This means that nursing care is dependent upon the accurate and unique assessment of the patient's need. As such this is an individual process but this section will identify some common areas of problem.

A patient will have one or more of cognitive, sensory or motor impairment. The accurate assessment of these impairments and appropriate responses will enable nurses to meet the needs of the patient. The contributors to this book have identified a range of post-stroke problems that will affect patients and also have identified appropriate responses. The potential problems are motor, sensory and cognitive dysfunction, but for all a consistent approach across the multi-disciplinary team is the most effective course of action. Nursing assessment may feed into other therapists' plans as well as the nursing diagnosis. Nursing practice will continue the work of other therapists as well as its own practices.

Intake of water or food

Following a stroke the patient may have been unable to drink or eat for a number of hours. This plus 'nil by mouth' nursing practices related to concerns over the patient's ability to swallow may facilitate potential dehydration and malnutrition. As a stroke may affect the competency of the swallow reflex, the patient's ability to swallow must be assessed before they eat or drink. The speech and language therapist is the optimal person for this assessment, especially if there is any doubt. Nurses and doctors are able to assess but should receive instruction in this process from speech and language therapists. If the swallow reflex is competent, then a normal feeding regimen should be instigated which should encompass the likely increased metabolic requirements. This assessment of the swallow reflex should be done as part of the admission process.

Fluids

An accurate assessment of the patient's need for fluids can be made from their blood electrolyte levels. An indication can also be obtained from their history, skin elasticity and urine output. Following a stroke, patients usually require at least 2–3 litres of fluid per day, which may be higher than their normal intake. The intention is to compensate for any slight dehydration, ensure sufficient fluid for homeostasis and to prevent constipation (Venn *et al.*, 1992).

Constipation may result from a reduction in peristalsis due to altered autonomic stimulation of the bowel and less exercise. If the stool remains longer in the bowel, then more fluid will be absorbed from the large bowel making the stool harder and more difficult to pass. This will result in increased intracranial pressure and discomfort, both of which are detrimental to the patient (Hickey, 1997). It is vital to assess the patient's need and their ability to meet that need by oral intake. If they are unable to meet the need, then either enteral (via a nasogastric tube) or parenteral (intravenously) feeding must be evaluated and the appropriate measures taken. The nurse must monitor and record fluid intake and output and provide encouragement, information and support for patients in achieving an adequate fluid intake.

Nutrition

Damage to the brain following a stroke will impact on the nutritional needs of the patient. Clifton *et al.* (cited by Woodward, 1996) demonstrated in 1984 that the resting metabolic expenditure was 260% of normal in a head injured person. The three factors found to be predictive of resting metabolic expenditure in the first two weeks post-injury were: (1) Glasgow Coma Score, (2) heart rate and (3) the number of days since injury (Woodward, 1996). Failure to address the increased nutritional needs of the post-stroke patient will lead to malnutrition, which will inhibit healing and the recovery of function (Torrance, 1990). A high protein/calorie diet is usually appropriate, as is the use of dietary supplements to achieve the patient's estimated dietary needs. The dietician is the optimal person to determine nutritional need and advise on methods to achieve it.

If the patient is unable to swallow adequately, then two approaches are available: either enteral or parenteral feeding. Enteral feeding has the advantage of using the digestive system as normal and the use of higher fibre feeds helps prevent the problem of constipation with its potential for raising intracranial pressure. Twyman *et al.* (1985) demonstrated that tube displacement and poor absorption can lead to abdominal distension, aspiration pneumonia and diarrhoea. Norton *et al.* (1988) showed that the lower the Glasgow Coma Score, the longer it took to tolerate enteral feeding.

Endacott (1993) showed that parenteral feeding ran increased risks of pneumothorax, embolism, infection and fluid and electrolyte imbalances. Waters *et al.* (1986, cited in Woodward, 1996) suggested that intravenous feeding may be linked to increasing cerebral oedema. However, the study by Rapp *et al.*, 1983 (cited by Woodward, 1996) demonstrated that parenteral nutrition led to better immunocompetence and prevented early death.

In summary, it appears that parenteral nutrition is likely to be tolerated earlier in the stroke patient; and although enteral feeding will be tolerated, the more extensive the brain damage, then the greater is the indication for parenteral nutrition. However, enteral nutrition is effective and is easier to manage both in general wards and in the home. What appears to be most important is the need to accurately assess the person's nutritional needs and to commence feeding as soon after admission as possible. As Nyswonger & Helmchen (1992) demonstrate, commencing feeding within 72 hours of admission significantly reduces the time spent in hospital.

The nurse's role in relation to nutrition is: to seek appropriate information and advice; to plan and carry out care appropriate to need; to monitor the patient's food and fluid intake and ensure that they satisfy the patient's need; to ensure that feeding does begin within 72 hours of admission and in a manner appropriate to needs.

Eliminative functions

Bowels

Normal control of bowel function is mediated through two systems. Firstly, the parasympathetic nervous system stimulates peristaltic waves and increased motility throughout the intestines. This response is strongest about 30 minutes after ingesting food. Secondly, stretch receptors in the rectum stimulate a spinal arc reflex to void, when distended. This reflex is normally mediated by the cerebrum to allow involvement of other parts of the body (constriction of chest and abdominal muscles and slight raising of knees) to raise intra-abdominal pressure. It also allows defecation to take place at a socially acceptable time and place. The reflex can also be artificially induced by raising the intra-abdominal pressure through the patient sitting on the toilet with the feet on a support so that the knees are raised slightly above the hips or by digital stimulation (Hickey, 1997; Munchiando & Kendall, 1993).

Normal patterns of defecation can vary from more than once daily to once every five days. Alterations to that pattern can lead to feelings akin to diarrhoea (if too often) and fullness, abdominal discomfort, loss of appetite and nausea (if not often enough). The ideal is that the person should be able to pass a soft, fully formed stool, without discomfort in a pattern with which they are comfortable. Following a stroke the person may lose awareness of the stretch receptors in the rectum or have difficulty altering their intra-abdominal pressure to initiate defecation. This 'loss of control' can lead to feelings of shame, dirtiness and loss of independence (Benson, 1975, cited in Munchiando & Kendall, 1993).

Venn *et al.* (1992) demonstrated that stroke patients tend to fall below the recommended daily intake of fibre (20–35g) and fluid (1500–3000ml). Also that achievement of these levels seemed to make successful bowel control easier. However, the strongest stimulants to normal defecation seemed to be eating and exercise. Daily use of suppositories, increasing to soap and water enemas if defecation did not follow, enables predictable daily defecation in two weeks with most patients.

The nurse's role in relation to bowel management for patients with strokes is the prevention of problems (primarily constipation) in a manner that optimizes patient control and comfort. As such it is about determining what is normal for the patient and monitoring what is actually happening at present. As the strongest stimulants to normal bowel control are food, fluid and exercise, then it is important to ensure that enough of each is taken by the patient. If faeces remain longer in the bowel than would be normal, then more water will be absorbed from it, making the stool harder and more difficult to pass. To avoid this problem high-fibre diets should be instigated to retain water in the faeces along with a daily fluid intake of at least 2000ml. As peristalsis is at a maximum 30 minutes after eating, then smaller, more frequent meals should encourage more peristalsis by increasing the amount of maximum peristalsis (the smaller meals are often more appealing to the patient and seem more manageable). Bolus feeding of naso-gastric feeds encourages greater peristalsis, as opposed to continuous feeding. The rehabilitation process and the exercise involved will help promote normal bowel activity as well as promoting the return of limb function – therefore, promotion of rehabilitation as soon as possible after the stroke will also promote bowel management. Positioning the patient when using the toilet can also help, i.e. providing a foot stool so that the knees are slightly raised above the hips to increase intra abdominal pressure. If control of the bowel cannot be achieved through these more normal mechanisms, then the nurse has to restore the patient's control through artificial means, such as manual evacuations, the use of suppositories and laxatives/apperients (Venn *et al.*, 1992 and Munchiando & Kendall, 1993).

Urinary incontinence

Urinary continence is a person's ability to void urine in socially acceptable places, at socially acceptable times in socially acceptable ways. It is also the ability to retain urine for at least twenty minutes until those socially acceptable situations exist. As such urinary continence is a learnt behaviour determined by the society within which the person lives.

Normal control of micturition involves coordinated activity within the frontal lobe, pons variola and the spinal cord (levels S2–S4 & T9–L2). Stretch receptors in the bladder stimulate the brain of the need to micturate, the greater the stretch, the stronger the stimulus. The hypothalamus and the medial frontal cortex determine the behaviour associated with micturition and can inhibit voiding until an acceptable situation is found (normally for about twenty minutes). In the dorsal pons, the medial pontine region (MPR) controls bladder contraction and the lateral pontine region (LPR) controls the sphincters. A coordinated response between these centres controls voiding:

Stimulate MPR & Inhibit LPR = Voiding urine

Inhibit MPR & Stimulate LPR = Not voiding urine

In the spinal cord, between levels S2 and S4, are the nuclei for the sensory and motor nerves controlling the bladder and sphincters. The S2–S4 supply is parasympathetic in nature and primarily involved in bladder contraction. The hypogastric nerve (T9–L2) is the sympathetic nerve supply to the bladder and it relaxes the bladder muscles. A spinal arc reflex will initiate voiding if the stretch receptors are excessively stretched. Eventually the reflex response will override cerebral and/or pontine control. This reflex arc will initiate voiding. The process is less coordinated than pontine control so voiding is liable to be incomplete (Lindsay *et al.*, 1995; Hickey, 1997; Cohen, 1999).

Strokes can affect different parts of the nervous system controlling normal micturition. Successful management of urinary incontinence will depend upon an accurate assessment of the problem. The assessment needs to consider: when and where voiding takes place, how much is voided, personal awareness, attitude and desire, any residual urine, any dribbling, the appropriateness and availability of toilet facilities, personal mobility and sensation, the amount of time the person has before voiding takes place, and the smell of the urine. The nature of the assessment means that the process is ongoing and will take time but as patterns become apparent appropriate measures can be taken (O'Connor, 1993; Gibbon, 1994; Hickey, 1997).

A catheter may have been inserted whilst the patient is in the acute stage and/ or unconscious. This should be removed as soon as possible, to allow assessment of any problem and to prevent a urinary tract infection developing (Cochran *et al.*, 1994; Hickey, 1997).

Palpate or percuss the bladder during the assessment period to indicate the presence of residual urine. Cystometry may provide information of the reflex state of the bladder. If large volumes of residual urine are present after voiding then intermittent catheterisation is indicated. With good technique this procedure is less socially disruptive and less likely to cause a urinary tract infection than long term catheterisation. Most problems of retention in stroke patients however will resolve within two weeks (Moore, 1994; Bannister, 1994; Cochran *et al.*, 1994).

Repetitive contraction of the pelvic muscles will help to develop muscle tone and prevent incontinence. Repeated contraction and then relaxation (about 10 seconds each) of the anal sphincter and perivaginal muscles (Kagel exercises) without stimulating other muscle groups will develop micturition control for women in about 4–6 weeks. The more the practice the better the effect, but a minimum of 50–100 exercises must be done daily to be effective. For men stopping and starting the stream helps to develop sphincter control (Long *et al.*, 1995; Hickey, 1997).

If the detruser muscle is 'unstable' then medication such as oxybutynin chloride may help prevent incontinence (Karch, 1999). Antibiotics or antifungals will treat any urinary tract infection present. The person must be aware that bladder sensation can be disrupted by a stroke and that the time they have to resist voiding can be reduced. The person also needs to be able to physically reach appropriate toilet facilities within their timescale. Assessment by a physiotherapist and/or occupational therapist may help identify aids or exercises relevant to the person's needs. Bottles, bedpans, commodes and/or location to toilet facilities needs to be considered when planning patient care (Bannister, 1992; Gibbon, 1994; Hickey, 1997).

If the assessment reveals a pattern of a loss of social control then behavioural approaches to treatment are relevant. This is a process of relearning socially acceptable behaviour through education, routinising behaviour and positively rewarding good behaviour. The person needs to understand what is going on and why. They need to identify their desired state and how in cooperation with their carers they can achieve that goal. Education and understanding help everyone to effectively work together to help achieve the desired outcome.

Following a stroke and with adequate hydration, the person should be voiding urine every 2–3 hours. The person may be reminded and/or checked for dryness every 2–4 hours. Inhibiting the sensation of a full bladder may involve delaying voiding for increasing times to the normal 20 minutes. This when balanced with adjusting the fluid load will increase bladder volume and help restore normal control.

Appropriate behaviour and positive results need to be re inforced to encourage that behaviour. Appropriate praise should be given consistently, but exaggerated praise can be counterproductive. Normal communication needs to be maintained throughout, whether attempts to improve the person's continence are successful or not. Negative responses to behaviour may encourage poor behaviour especially in the presence of limited normal communication (Oates *et al.*, cited in Bancroft & Carr, 1995; Hickey, 1997). Appropriate praise and recognition of results will help the person through providing a psychological boost. Improvements in continence will also help restore the person's confidence to re-enter social situations (Gibbon, 1994).

Activity balanced with rest

Positioning

As demonstrated in Chapter 6, all stroke patients require an individualized approach to meeting their unique needs during the process of regaining motor control. Physiotherapists, as 'the only hands-on profession whose core expertise is designed to promote the rehabilitation or restoration of physical movement and ability', are essential in providing some care and advising others. However, their input is limited due to time and workload constraints, usually to a maximum of an 'hour or so, daily at first'. As such, much of this care is continued by nurses and/or relatives and is most effective when carried out in liaison with the physiotherapist. The rehabilitation process to be effective must begin with admission/diagnosis and be directed at meeting the individual's unique needs and be continued consistently 24 hours a day (Tyson, 1995). This section will discuss some nursing considerations in relation to positioning the patient that should be considered when determining the care plan.

Venous return to the heart from the brain is increased when the person is nursed at 30 degrees as opposed to lying flat (Hickey, 1997). Lippe & Mitchell (1980) cited in Rising (1993) also showed that flexion, extension and twisting of the neck reduced venous return. Inhibition of venous return increases the amount of blood retained within the 'brain'. This reduces the pressure gradient between the cerebral tissues and the venous system, which promotes the retention of fluid in the cerebral tissues (oedema) and raises the intracranial pressure. To maintain the cerebral perfusion pressure, the blood pressure must consequently rise, but this may prove detrimental to the management of the acute stroke patient. With the patient lying flat, blood pressure is lower, as the heart does not have to compete with gravity but the venous return is reduced. However, lying flat encourages a more passive patient role, as it is more difficult to be active (to eat or drink independently), and this is liable to cause frustration which with stress, pain and anxiety will raise the intracranial pressure (Hickey, 1997).

Nursing the patient at 30 degrees proves beneficial by minimizing cerebral oedema and improving patient comfort. This is ideally done on a bed, which raises the patient on the mattress rather than using a backrest and pillows. This makes it easier to adjust the patient's angle and reduces the risk of pressure damage to the skin through breaks in the pillow support. This position also makes it easier to correctly position the patient in relation to their stroke and maintain their comfort. At all times the head and neck should be supported so that a straight alignment is maintained, which requires the use of pillows depending on the individual's size and the size of the pillows (Carr & Kennedy, 1992). Positioning the person's limbs is designed to prevent spasticity by promoting 'reflex inhibiting' patterns of posture (Carr & Kennedy, 1992). Appropriate use of these positions will maintain tissue viability and promote rehabilitation.

To inhibit pressure sore damage patients should ideally not be nursed on their backs, but on alternate sides at 30 degrees to vertical. This means that pressure is applied to more 'padded areas', rather than directly over bony areas (sacrum, etc.). When rolling the patient, nurses should treat the affected limbs as fragile and use the scapula and the hip as the places to apply kinetic energy. Pulling on the person's affected arm may lead to dislocation of the shoulder.

Passive exercises of the affected limb can be done each time the patient is repositioned to help prevent spasticity. This involves gently moving the joints through their normal range of movements, but when the limb is raised against gravity the joints must be supported by the nurse and the range of movements applied must never overextend the joint so that dislocation occurs. The extent of these exercises can be reduced at night to promote sleep but should not be excluded. However, if night exercising cannot be done, then the exercising in the day should be more extensive and should be carried out in a pattern agreed with the physiotherapist. This activity will help prevent spasticity, will promote the venous return from the limbs (especially the leg) and provide a more normal sleep/wake/activity pattern.

Rest

Torrance (1990) links sleep and food intake with increased tissue repair and suggests that REM sleep (rapid eye movement) may be particularly linked to the restoration of brain tissues, whilst orthodox sleep is more related to the restoration of body tissues. Adequate rest also promotes the patient's psychological well-being and facilitates their ability to deal with the stroke.

Hospitals and illness are not conducive to a normal sleep pattern. Strange environments, people and noises as well as alterations in the person's normal activity and stimulation will affect their sleeping pattern. Napping during the day and difficulty in sleeping at night may make the person feel psychologically unfit, even though over the 24-hour period they have managed their normal amount of sleep.

The nurse's role is to facilitate a normal sleep pattern by finding out how long the person normally sleeps, between what hours and how rested they feel after their sleep. Are there any practices/processes that they normally undertake prior to sleep? What and how much activity do they undertake during the day? The level of the patient's consciousness will influence their sleeping pattern, but the nurse needs to develop an activity/rest cycle conducive to that person's needs. Following a stroke patients are likely to have an increased need for sleep, so nurses should plan daily activities to include adequate rest periods and sufficient stimulation/activity to induce a 'good nights sleep' and the recovery of function. As the needs of each individual are unique and are liable to change over a period of hospitalization, practice and procedures need to be evaluated daily and appropriate changes instigated (Hickey, 1997).

Being alone and being with others

When a person has had a stroke, the days immediately following (when they usually require most rest) often coincide with the time when most friends and family wish to see them. Restrictions at this time upon the range of visitors and the length of their stay are liable to prove beneficial to the patient. As the patient's condition improves, fixed visiting times can become a problem because visitors may feel that they have to stay for the fixed period; but the patient's limited range of stimuli may mean that their contribution to any conversation becomes stilted and the visiting period may become awkward for all. Fixed visiting times also tend to discourage family/friends/partners' participation and involvement in the rehabilitation process. Visiting times need to be flexible to fit in with the visitors' and the patient's daily life and for both not to feel guilty about having shorter visits. This flexibility also facilitates teaching the patient and their appropriate family/friends/partner about appropriate rehabilitation practices and processes.

The stroke patient also needs time alone to reflect on events and determine how they will face the change in their lives. They are likely to encounter some, if not all, of the various stages of grief as defined by Kubler-Ross, 1969 (cited in Gormley & Brodzinsky, 1989) – namely denial, anger, bargaining, depression and acceptance. These stages will influence the person's input into their rehabilitation process. The nurse is able to listen, talk, educate, encourage, cajole and support the person's rehabilitation; but in the end the patient must take charge of their own recovery.

The nurse should have an open relationship with the patient which is based on trust – to observe verbal and non-verbal clues about the patient's need for company; to be available if needed but not to force interaction unless a patient's desire to be alone hinders rehabilitation. The patient needs to determine whom they see, for how long and, within reason, when – they also have the right to be alone but not to be isolated.

In the post-hospital stage patients require even greater social support. Many stroke patients on returning home may be independent but differently able. They may be able to walk but are not as quick or are less sure of themselves. About a third of people with strokes suffer a degree of depression, and so difficulties with their normal social and work interactions may lead to withdrawal. Motivation from family and friends to return to old interests or develop new ones is essential in restoring the patient to their optimal state of health – not only to help physical recovery but also to promote social and psychological health. It is essential for the nurse to encourage the family and friends to take a supportive role (Tyson, 1995).

Being alone

Being alone does not mean that a person is isolated. People have a need to reflect upon situations and so determine their course of action. Being continually stimulated will prevent rest and inhibit the person in coming to terms with their stroke. The provision of exercises to restore function, which can be done alone, promotes the restoration of function and may also focus the person's mind. The nurse's role is to enable the person to be alone when they wish but to prevent isolation. To this end they must ensure that the patient knows that the nurse is available and that they have the means to call him or her. The nurse should also observe body language and offer opportunities for the patient to talk or seek company as and when they desire. Although some people will express a wish to be alone but will really seek communication, most, if not all, people will at times need to be alone (Hickey, 1997).

Needing carers

The family/friends of a patient diagnosed with a stroke will undergo a host of emotions such as anger, loss, guilt, fear, frustration and confusion. The intensity of these emotions will depend upon the nature of their relationship with the patient, and this is impossible to pre-judge. Coping with a patient's disability may prove harder for the family/friends than coping with the patient's death (Rosenthal *et al.*, 1993). As the family/friends are an essential part of the rehabilitation process, it is part of the nurse's role to be aware of their problems and needs.

The emotional state of the family/friends will be compounded by their lack of knowledge and may also inhibit their learning process. As such, information needs to be given in appropriate ways – in honest, short and manageable pieces which reflect the stated needs of the family/friends. Understanding can be assessed with questioning from the nurse, and simple explanations can be expanded as the person deals with the information. The person, though, who directs the spread of information remains the patient.

Family/friends will wish to know things like: What can they do to help the patient? What will the patient be able to do and by when? How can they be involved in the care? What care is being given and why? They will also wish to be treated with honesty, to feel that there is hope and to be involved in any plans and decisions (Rosenthal *et al.*, 1993). Involving the family/friends in the patient's care helps them to learn what the patient can and cannot do and how they can safely adapt, identify potential problems and be involved in finding solutions. This involvement will help spread understanding and assist family/friends in dealing with the patient's stroke, thereby easing their emotional responses to the stroke and reducing potential anxieties for everyone involved. The involvement of family/friends in the rehabilitation process assists in the preparation for the patient's discharge.

References

Aggleton, P. & Chalmers, H. (1986) *Nursing Models and the Nursing Process*. Macmillan, London.

Bancroft, D. & Carr, R. (1995) In *Influencing Children's Development* (J. Oates, M. Hoghughi & R. Dallas, eds), pp. 277–313. The Open University, Milton Keynes.

Bannister, R. (1992) *Brain and Bannister's Clinical Neurology*. Oxford University Press, Oxford.

Carr, E.K. & Kennedy, F.D. (1992) Positioning of the stroke patient: a review of the literature. *International Journal of Nursing Studies* **4**(29/11), 355–69.

Chinn, P. & Kramer, M. (1991) *Theory and Nursing: A Systematic Approach*. Mosby Year Book, St Louis.

Cochran, I., Flynn, C.A., Goetz, G., Potts-Nulty, S.E., Rece, J. & Sensenig, H. (1994) In the literature. Stroke care: piecing together the long term picture. *Nursing* **24**, 34–41.

Cohen, H. (1999) *Neuroscience for Rehabilitation*. Lippincott Williams and Wilkins, Philadelphia.

Endacott, R. (1993) Nutritional support for critically ill patients. *Nursing Standard* **7**(15), 25–8.

Frawley, P. (1990) Neurological observations. *Nursing Times* **86**(35), 29–32.

Gibbon, B. (1994) Stroke care and rehabilitation. *Nursing Standard* **8**(33), 49–54.

Gormley, A. & Brodzinsky, D. (1989) *Lifespan Human Development.* Holt, Rhinehart and Winston Inc., London.

Hickey, J.V. (1997) *The Clinical Practice of Neurological and Neurosurgical Nursing*, 4th edn., Lippincott, New York.

Karch, A. (1999) *Lippincott's Nursing Drug Guide.* Lippincott Williams and Wilkins, Philadelphia.

Lindsay, K., Bone, I. & Callander, R. (1995) *Neurology and Neurosurgery Illustrated*, 2nd Edn. Churchill Livingstone, London.

Long, B.C., Phipps, W.J. & Cassmeyer, V.C. (1995) *Adult Nursing: A nursing process approach.* Mosby, London.

McCaffery (1979) *Nursing Management of Patients in Pain* 2nd edn. J.B. Lippincott, Philadelphia.

Moore, K. (1994) Stroke: the long road back. *Rehabilitation Nursing* March, 50–54.

Munchiando, J. & Kendall, K. (1993) Comparison of the effectiveness of two bowel programmes for CVA patients. *Rehabilitation Nursing* **18**(3), 168–72.

Norton, J., Orr, L., McClain, C. & Adams, L. (1988) Intolerance of enteral feeding in the brain injured patient. *Journal of Neurosurgery* **68**, 62–6.

Nyswonger, G. & Helmchen, R. (1992) Early enteral nutrition and length of stay in stroke patients. *Journal of Neuroscience Nursing* **4**(24), 220–23.

O'Connor, S.E. (1993) Nursing and rehabilitation: the interventions in stroke patient care. *Journal of Clinical Nursing* **2**, 29–34.

Rising, C. (1993) The relationship of selected nursing activities to ICP. *Journal of Neuroscience Nursing* **25**(5), 302–18.

Rosenthal, S., Pituch, M., Greninger, L. & Metress, E. (1993) Perceived needs of wives of stroke patients. *Rehabilitation Nursing* **18**(3), 148–53, 167, 207–18.

Rowley, G. & Fielding, K. (1991) Reliability and accuracy of the Glasgow Coma Scale with experienced and inexperienced users. *The Lancet* **337**(8740), 535–8.

Segatore, M. (1996) Understanding central post-stroke pain. *Journal of Neuroscience Nursing* **28**(1), 28–35.

Shepard, T.J. & Fox, S.W. (1996) Assessment and management of hypertension in the acute ischaemic stroke patient. *Journal of Neuroscience Nursing* **28**(1), 5–12.

Torrance, C. (1990) Sleep and wound healing. *Surgical Nurse* 3(3), 16–20.

Tortora, G. & Anagnostakos, N. (1990) *Principles of Anatomy and Physiology*, 6th edn. Harper Collins Publishers, New York.

Twyman, D., Young, B. & Ott, L.G. (1985) High protein enteral feeding: a means of achieving positive nitrogen balance in head injured patients. *Journal of Parenteral/Enteral Nutrition* **9**(6), 679–84.

Tyson, S.F. (1995) Stroke rehabilitation: what is the point? *Physiotherapy* **81**(8), 430–32.

Venn, M.R., Taft, L., Carpentier, B. & Applebaugh, G. (1992) The influence of timing and suppository use on efficiency and effectiveness of bowel training after a stroke. *Rehabilitation Nursing* **17**(3), 36–41.

Woodward, S. (1996) Nutritional support for head-injured patients. *Professional Nurse* **11**(5), 44–8.

Chapter 5

Enable or Disable: Evidence-Based Clinical Problem-Solving

Polly Laidler

A stroke strikes at the source of all activity and will always result in residual problems of varying severity – not merely as the result of the localized brain cell destruction but also because this creates a 'glitch' in the infinitely complex and multilevel networking systems of the brain. The site of a neural lesion does not necessarily correlate directly with the loss of a specific function (Hertanu *et al.*, 1984). A lesion in the same anatomically located area of the brain in another stroke survivor does not produce the same set of problems in both people, and it is unwise to generalize between the effects of apparently obvious right and left hemisphere damage; the dominant hemisphere is seldom the right in left-handed people, for instance.

We all possess uniquely constructed brain cell systems formed from the accumulation of inherited/genetic structure in conjunction with individually acquired skills and behavioural responses due to environmental influences in addition to special differences – physical, metabolic, specific numerical, artistic or musical talents – and to cognitive anomalies such as dyslexia.

Therefore, any focal lesion will produce a subtly differing range of disabilities (each of which are quite likely to respond differently to intervention) in every adult human being; and because of this it is unrealistic to expect standard formulae for problem-solving. Any apparently common-to-many impairments are accrued from diverse sources and will each require in-depth assessment and a diversity of treatment approaches.

Functional capability may appear to depend largely on physical ability, but the ability to move body and limbs has nothing to do with their actual usefulness in the performance of even simple tasks: the 'loss of use' of one arm and/or one leg will create mechanical difficulties but seldom prevents the practical re-adjustments necessary for the continuation of competent functional activity or the return to a relatively normal way of life.

As a stroke produces neurological disorganization, the diminished functional ability after a stroke is the result of:

(1)   Cognitive and perceptual impairment
(2)   Sensory and motor impoverishment
(3)   Uninhibited reflex activity
(4)   Altered tonicity

The last two factors, when reinforced by subsequent ineffectively managed neurological reorganization, result in hyper-reflexia and spasticity. Recovery, 'good' or 'poor', is the result of neurological reorganization.

Interdisciplinary teamwork, the collaborative approach, held together by a common-core thread of specialized knowledge, is the essential element in neurorehabilitation. This well-accepted doctrine is not always fully implemented in clinical practice, possibly because 'the Reason Why' has remained heuristic. However, the quality and quantity of neuroscientific evidence now accumulating confirms that the traditional linear approach to stroke rehabilitation can, in fact, prove to be inadvert. Professional intervention has, in many instances, been further disabling rather than enabling for the stroke survivor. It would seem that our approach to problem-solving has been rooted in misconceptions about the origin of these problems: we have been treating the symptoms rather than the cause. It is the quality of the input that counts, not merely the quantity.

This chapter collates the evidence as a baseline to reconstruct the rehabilitation process in relation to stroke; it links cause with effect for informed problem-solving and discusses the implications for recovery and rehabilitation. Two fundamental issues that contribute to many of the problems which may be experienced after a stroke are reviewed briefly first.

Neuromuscular plasticity

Plasticity in this context is the ability of cells to alter any aspect of their phenotype (gene characteristic), at any stage in development, in response to abnormal changes in their state of environment (Brown & Hardman, 1987).

Muscle fibres are polymorphic and respond entirely to demand. Ten percent of muscle protein changes daily, molecule by molecule (Kidd *et al.*, 1992); catabolism (atrophy) and anabolism (hypertrophy) are directed by the decrease or increase in protein synthesis.

Motor neurons respond to any significant change in physical activity via the terminal synapse (neuromuscular endplate), and the changing protein synthesis in the peripheral nerve tissue is transmitted to the higher centres of the central nervous system (CNS). If the same action is repeated often enough, the bombardment of identical stimuli initiates the growth of new dendrites (in the Purkinje cell in the cerebellum, for instance) to link with other nerve cell endings to form new – or to strengthen existing – synapses, networks and pathways. Receptors are built as required and lost when not required. New synapses evolve in seven days and are strengthened by frequent usage.

Repetition of identical stimuli for long enough to produce positive change in the neuromuscular system is known as physiological stressing. A clear example is the way cardiac muscle responds to consistent exercise training by slowing its pumping rate to enable prolonged strenuous activity without exhaustion: this change in rate is controlled by the ability of the CNS to change its output in response to changing demands.

When there has been focal cell destruction, of course, there can be no cell restructuring. No soma = no plasticity. This accounts for the apparent loss of certain elements of speech, memory and movement after a stroke.

Any type of movement performed has a transient effect on existing networks. If it is repeated over a significant period of time, then plastic adaptation of the neuromuscular system ensures that it becomes part of the library of motor behaviour for reproduction in all relevant situations. This applies whether the movement is involuntary or volitional, 'normal' or distorted, assisted, resisted or free (Laidler, 1994).

Physiological adaptation takes only days to become established. It is a continuous process, and is a hugely significant factor affecting recovery from the moment of brain trauma onwards. Given the plasticity of the neuromuscular system, physiological stressing can make possible the restructuring of near-normal movement patterns (taking into account any residual focal loss). It can also, however, build abnormal motor behaviour.

The implications for recovery and rehabilitation are obvious. Stereotyped reflexes, spasticity, abnormal movement patterns, over-compensatory movements, non-use of the hemiplegic limbs, and even dependency on physical help from others – these are physiologically programmed to become the 'normal' structured responses to stimulation – hardwired into the system to be reproduced automatically in response to the need to move. They are the secondary, acquired disabilities.

Where the lesion has formed an irreparable obstacle within the acquired information processing systems, alternative networks can in many cases be established to produce a useful level of functional activity (Bach-y-Rita, 1981; Bishop, 1982).

Cognitive control of movement

The developments in this neuroscientific field have to influence our approach to rehabilitation. Bate (1997) summarizes the motor control theories which she categorizes into two broad groups: 'Information Processing' and 'Action' (interaction between the organism and the environment) theories, as discussed later in this chapter.

For the second fundamental issue in this section, Mulder's 'process-oriented model of human motor control' is described and then followed up with a closer look at the more common problems experienced by many stroke survivors, such as cognitive and perceptual impairment.

Motor behaviour is the result of the integrated activity of a complex system consisting of many parallel information transforming processes. Mulder (1993) has collated recent studies into a computational model (illustrated in Fig. 5.1).

To perform an action, an optimal level of activation is necessary. Exhaustion, alcohol, coma, and certain drugs, for instance, lower the arousal level to such a degree that the organism is no longer able to respond adequately to stimuli. All normal movements are performed to meet a perceived need or goal. This

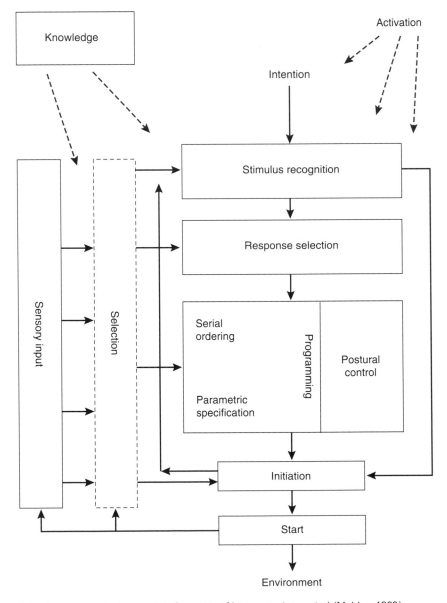

Fig. 5.1 A process-oriented model of aspects of human motor control (Mulder, 1993).

'intention' activates a stored repertoire of rules or 'action schemata' (Epstein, 1986).

The nervous system is subjected to a continuous bombardment of internal and external stimuli, much of which is likely to be irrelevant for the particular act to be performed. Selection of relevant information is therefore crucial to filter out the non-essential stimuli. Without this process every bit of data would have the same value and the same potential to trigger a reaction, resulting in chaotic motor activity.

To determine the relevance of stimuli, they have to be identified. Recognition of relevant stimuli is part of this selection process and dependent upon memory. It is not a conscious memory search but the exploitation of tacit knowledge (Klein, 1976; Wise & Desimone, 1988; Reber, 1989). For example, the significance of a ringing telephone has to be known in order for it to be dealt with appropriately. Many of the agnosias (loss of recognition of familiar objects) which result in disturbed functional competence are due to disruption in this area.

The theory of the motor response is now expanded from the traditional concept of almost infinite sets of pre-programmed motor engrams to allow for the subtle interaction between knowledge and movement. Motor learning, like language, is now thought to require the acquisition of a limited set of schemata or 'programming rules' – a library of prototypes in more abstract form – which together create a 'grammar of action' which functions as the interface between cognition and action. This is a significant factor with far reaching implications for rehabilitation.

Programming of a motor response is therefore the construction of *ad hoc* motor programmes on the basis of acquired rules in conjunction with information selected from the environment. It comprises at least two subprocesses: serial ordering, the sequential order of movements needed to perform the required activity; and parametric specification, the addition of task- and context-specific information, such as the force and direction needed for the task, to the motor programme under construction. Disorder in these processes produces ideational dyspraxias and anomalies in spatial judgement.

Anticipatory postural mechanisms are alerted by perceptual and sensory input to allow for disturbances in relation to gravity. This series of computational processes ends with the actual initiation of the movement. Cross-referencing by feedback and feedforward at all times between all levels is necessary for any movement to be performed efficiently. This allows for the alterations in movement if the goal or environment itself changes after the movement is initiated, as in swerving to avoid an unforeseen hazard or catching a tipping cup.

No clear separation exists between the sensory, cognitive and motor mechanisms in the construction of a response. 'Normal movement' is not just a neuromuscular response to stimulation, it is the result of dynamic interaction between cognitive and motor skills. A stroke creates havoc in this complex networking and can disrupt all human activity.

Cognitive and perceptual impairment

These deficits produce the invisible problems of stroke, in that the physical ability to perform a movement can be unaffected (as with apparently good recovery of movement in the hemiplegic limbs) but the performance of even basic tasks may be jeopardized, flawed, or impossible.

Cognitive impairment as a result of a stroke is just that: the intellect remains unchanged but the ability to direct mind over matter is faulty. It is often mistaken for a deterioration in 'intelligence' and can be mislabelled as confusion or even dementia particularly in older clients, which could influence all future intervention. For any adult, such a drastic misunderstanding can be a major factor affecting outcome and also contribute to severe depression.

With informed guidance and rehabilitation many of the cognitive deficits can be modified, if not overcome. Although full independence may not be achieved in all cases (some people will always require a carer to provide the necessary cueing for activity), quality of life should always be dramatically improved. There is an infinite variety of these non-visible but extremely disabling problems, caused by a lesion that interferes with cognitive processing or actually obstructs access to vital databanks in the brain.

Dyspraxia

Dyspraxia is the inability to perform certain purposeful movements even though motor power and sensation may be normal. It is frequently associated with dominant hemisphere lesions, so communication can be further impoverished with this articulatory and gestural hazard. Of all the dyspraxias identified to date, the two most commonly seen and diagnosed are 'ideomotor' and 'ideational'. Ideomotor dyspraxia is a constructional disorder: an impairment in the selection of components of a functional movement (relating to 'response selection' in Mulder's model as illustrated in Fig. 5.1).

The performance of even simple tasks to command is impossible even with the unaffected limbs. People with this dyspraxia will say (if language is not compromised by dysphasia), 'I know what you are asking me to do (e.g. get your feet off the wheelchair footplates) but I don't seem to be able to do it'. Teaching by verbal instruction, demonstration or physical assistance – to transfer between chairs, get in and out of garments, even to start walking, for instance – is not effective for these clients. However, in all cases automatic movement responses seem to be unimpaired, apart from some non-fluency of movement seen as a residual clumsiness or awkwardness. Given the appropriate cueing (subcortical stimulation), and by learning to respond instinctively to environmental clues, people with ideomotor dyspraxia are often able to achieve a fair level of independence.

Ideational dyspraxia is a conceptual disorder, an inability to carry out purposeful sequential acts either to command or automatically. (This corresponds to disorder in the 'serial ordering' component of programming in Mulder's model.) The stages of the movements and procedures are present but cannot be put together in the correct order. With this form of dyspraxia even 'automatic' movement responses cannot be prompted. As even the most simple tasks involve a complex sequencing of actions – washing, dressing, making a cup of tea – people with ideational dyspraxia are unlikely to achieve independence in many, if not all, functional activities unless spontaneous improvement occurs.

Unilateral neglect

Unilateral neglect is the ignoring of one-half of personal near and/or far space. Unlike hemianiopia it is not due to a visual field defect. Homonymous hemianopias (loss of one-half of the field of vision on the stroke side, affecting one or both eyes) following CVA are associated with lesions in the dominant hemisphere of the brain, usually with a right (R) sided hemiplegia. Clients with hemianopias quickly learn to scan to the affected side, using head movements in order to see into the 'missing' field of vision.

Unilateral neglect is particularly associated with lesions in the non-dominant hemisphere, so it is a frequent feature with a left (L) hemiplegia. People with this problem may not have any visual, sensory or motor impairment, but they still fail to respond, report or relate to stimuli presented to the stroke-affected side in both personal and extra-personal space. This has been described as 'impaired attentional or orienting systems' (Humphreys & Riddoch, 1987) and a 'disorder of representational schema' (Bisiach & Luzzatti, 1978).

This deficit presents with varying degrees of severity and can affect all activity, for example: all or part of the stroke-side (usually the left) of the face is left unshaved or without cosmetics; clothing and unclothing the stroke side of the body presents confusion; food on the left side of the plate may not be eaten; people and objects to the left of the client are not noticed; conversation coming from the left is ignored; reading and writing may be confined to the right side of every page; drawing and even copying simple drawings will leave areas incomplete on the left side of each item in the picture.

The degree of impoverishment in extrapersonal space often reflects the area of neglect in intrapersonal space: the missing bits of drawings may correlate with the same areas of unawareness of own-body geography as seen in the apparent denial of a stroke arm or the patchy problems in dressing, putting on make-up or shaving.

Rehabilitation has to refocus attention into this 'black hole' by the emphatic and repetitious use of visual stimuli. It is necessary to demand eye contact and work from midline into the unrecognized space. Clients need to add scanning to their repertoire of automatic skills, but many will never regain independence.

There is no evidence to date that memory itself can be restored with rehabilitation, but prospective memory can usually be worked on. Learning ability is unaffected if the 'working memory' is unimpaired. Self-help strategies can sometimes be learned, and much of the immediate environment can be adapted – colour-coding for toilet doors, for instance.

Agnosia

This is sensation without perception: the failure to recognize familiar objects, although the visual, tactile and auditory systems themselves are unimpaired. Like the dyspraxias, agnosia presents in various ways: visual (faces/places/things), tactile/touch (objects), and so on.

Case example: One stroke survivor was creating havoc on the ward at mealtimes. She tipped up everything from loaded dinnerplates to sugar bowls and cups of tea, and appeared to be deliberately choosing not to feed herself. She became increasingly aggressive, and a psychological assessment diagnosed dementia. Long-term care in the psychogeriatric unit (at the age of 57) was scheduled, to the obvious grief of her family (two sons with their own families) and her many friends. Her complete aphasia further complicated the issue, as did the fact that the therapists had found her to be enthusiastic and well-motivated in their own departments. A multidisciplinary assessment (to include the family) was finally arranged which began with a friendly cup of coffee in the physiotherapy department. She was discovered to have had a significant hearing loss as well as being aphasic and agnosic. Learning a gestural communication system based on Amer-Ind and encouragement to develop personal 'miming' improved her communication. She did not recognize the cup, for instance, until her hands were folded around it and guided to her mouth for drinking.

After a few weeks spent re-acquainting her with the objects encountered in all the activities of daily living, she became the darling of the ward, fetching and carrying and helping nurses to make beds and encouraging other stroke patients. She was soon confident enough to return to living alone in her own home, with a little support from family and friends (Laidler, 1994).

Disorientations in time and/or space

Like the agnosias, these actively influence functional ability. The confidence to utilize recovering motility is also affected.

Case example: A young woman turned up in a taxi at a local stroke unit accompanied by her mother. Her distress, which was compounded by a slight expressive dysphasia, needed immediate investigation. She had been housebound since a stroke six months earlier, diagnosed by her GP as 'mild' with a good recovery and therefore not referred for any assessment or rehabilitation, although on most days she seemed unable to walk about or cope with stairs.

She was discovered to be unable to differentiate between two- and three-dimensional outlines. For example, going up and down stairs was only possible if she didn't look at them, and as she had partially denervated musculature on her R side, with increasing hypertonicity in what remained, this was unrealistic for a start; if she looked at the lines of the treads, they just registered as two-dimensional straight lines as though flat on the floor. Having fallen badly several times, she was now too afraid to attempt the stairs. She found herself fearful of every move indoors: the edges of rugs and mats became new obstacles, thresholds and doorways with 'lines' between different carpets and rooms, loomed ominously.

Everyday life was a nightmare of hesitation, guesswork, decision-taking and disaster – shuffling, falling, groping and often reduced to crawling on hands and knees. Outdoors was terrifying: kerbs were indistinguishable from lines in the pavement, and road markings (double yellow lines and zebra crossings could be steps or stairs, up or down, no clues) so she faltered, tripped and/or fell even when walking arm-in-arm.

Her husband and teenage children had become impatient and neglectful, complaining about neurotic and attention-seeking behaviour. A suicide attempt brought in the psychiatric team and treatment for 'behavioural problems' as well as for depression.

For this client, a comforting explanation and the issue of an ordinary walking stick provided immediate salvation. The stick could be used discreetly to tap and sweep ahead of the feet to define flat surfaces and located steps up or down, and, if a step, the height or depth could be gauged against the stick. Sadly this remediation came too late to save her marriage and the relationship with one of her children (Laidler, 1994).

Anosognosia

This is a lack of comprehension of personal neurological deficit. If the lesion disrupts the area that organizes knowledge into reasoned thinking, no amount of explanation from others, however logical or repetitive, is going to link cause with effect. Clients with this problem are often labelled 'unrealistic'; they are, but it is unrealistic to expect them to be anything else. They can also be called 'unmotivated' for failing to comply with advice and do homework between therapy sessions; and many complain about lack of treatment because rehabilitation input is not recognized as treatment, as they cannot relate it to the problems arising from their stroke. Constantly requesting information and denying they have received any, these people can cause disruption and dissent among unwary members of a multidisciplinary team and anger and dismay in their own families.

They are not trouble-makers, they are frustrated – aware that they are beset by problems which they are desperately seeking to rationalize but unable to comprehend that the solutions remain beyond their understanding.

Sensory and motor impoverishment

Sensory impairment

The visual, auditory, tactile and proprioceptive sensory systems form the major afferent pathways conveying to the brain all the incoming information regarding self and the environment. We move in response to a need to move (see Fig. 5.2),

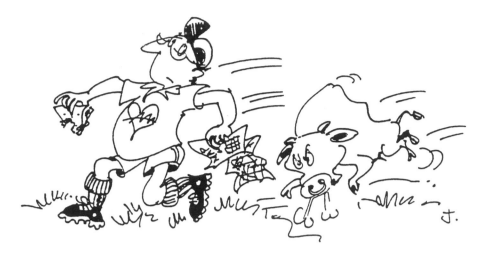

Fig. 5.2   We move in response to a need to move.

and a successful outcome is then dependent upon continuous feedback from the senses to monitor and correct ongoing performance in order to achieve the desired goal.

Where one or more sensory systems are impoverished or lost, the remaining senses become hyperactive in compensation. Visual impairment enhances tactile and proprioceptive faculties: reading braille, and stepping with a heightened sensitivity (for surface texture) and a shortened stride for safe walking are examples of this.

But the tactile and proprioceptive systems are those most commonly affected by a stroke. 'Lost' sensation is seldom fully recoverable; and therefore the recruitment of functional movement in the affected limbs (even where there is apparent 'recovery' of movement) demands total and continuous concentration plus visual feedback to initiate, sustain, and complete any activity. It is not surprising that clients with sensory deficits seem slow and 'unmotivated' to move. With no recognizable incoming sensory trigger, there can be no motor response. Trying to get up and walk with a leg that has 'gone to sleep', or to pick up a cup of tea using an upper limb deadened in the same way, makes one appreciate the full significance of this impairment! Many stroke survivors are elderly and/or diabetic with concomitant visual impoverishment and a generalized sensory 'dulling', which add to their difficulties. Eating and drinking can also be jeopardized.

The unaffected sensory systems need to be utilized in all rehabilitation strategies here, with vision allowed to take the primary role (i.e. 'don't keep looking down' is not practical advice).

Hypersensitivity

Occasionally the reception of tactile stimulation is intensified after a stroke. Even light brushing against the skin on the stroke side will produce a sharp searing or burning sensation that takes precedence over all else. This problem sometimes responds to desensitizing self-help strategies such as firm stroking or rubbing of the stroke limb using the non-stroke hand, to bombard the receptors until their excitability is overloaded.

Central post-stroke pain (CPSP)

In a few people another acute and ongoing hypersensitivity (formerly known as 'thalamic pain') develops some months after the stroke. It is present regardless of any actual contact with the skin; the receptors seem to switch on to Red Alert sending continuous pain and/or violent tingling signals, and the only respite is during sleep. Conventional painkilling drugs have no effect, neither do the transcutaneous electrical nerve stimulators (TENS) that interrupt the peripheral pain pathways – so daily life for these clients (who tend to present with a R hemiplegia and communication difficulties) is even more troubled.

Low doses of some of the 'first-generation' antidepressants such as amitriptyline, desipramine or mianserin (a tetracyclic) may alleviate the discomfort for some people after a month or so – not for depression but because these particular drugs help the higher centres of the brain to inhibit receptors in the spinal cord. The implanting of electrodes into the brain itself, for TENS-type transmitters carried externally, is possible now for otherwise intransigent cases and can be remarkably effective (Rawlings *et al.*, 1992).

Motor impairment

Impoverishment or loss of muscle innervation can result from direct loss of the coded cell structure at the site of the lesion. It is unusual for entire muscles to be blitzed in this way, but, if a large percentage of muscle fibres are denervated in a muscle, then the remainder may not give sufficient power to perform an adequate movement, particularly against the force of gravity. Physiological stressing has been known to stimulate new endplate activity and re-innervation, and it also makes possible the anabolism of non-affected muscle fibres to enhance their performance.

It is often only an apparent loss, due to a glitch in the information-processing systems in the CNS. Afferent signals may not be recognized, relevant data may be inaccessible; without cognitive control, purposeful movement is not possible. It is always essential to work through the battery of subcortical stimulation (detailed in the next chapter) to release 'automatic' movement responses in order to assess the situation correctly.

Uninhibited reflex activity

Stereotyped reflexes involve the primitive spinal cord patterns of movement in limbs and trunk. They are the ungraded responses (of flexion, extension, rotation) to a stimulus. They are total all-or-nothing reactions and as such are not part of any task-oriented activity.

A stroke disrupts the sophisticated control of these reflex patterns by the higher centres of the CNS. Disregulation of the complex interplay between inhibition and excitation leads to the traditional reflex reactions to stress or effort so frequently displayed by stroke survivors when trying to move. These reactions can also be precipitated by an active movement into any part of the reflex pattern.

The primitive reflex patterns include the positive supporting reflex (PSR) and the symmetrical and asymmetrical tonic neck reflexes: the positive supporting reflex is the 'push-down to push-off' reaction by foot and leg in response to pressure against the ball of the foot.

Rigid foot orthoses and footboards in beds (to support a 'dropped foot') will only reinforce this reflex and the problem. The foot is not 'dropped' as a result of flaccid musculature, it is in the grip of reflex activity which causes plantarflexion (and inversion, usually, too). The asymmetrical tonic neck reflex is demonstrated by turning the head to face sideways: this extends the arm to that side and flexes the arm on the other side.

For clients with this problem, walking with a stick used in the non-affected hand, elbow extended, will produce flexion in the stroke arm with the head pulled to face the non-stroke side.

The symmetrical tonic neck reflex is a response to flexion/extension of the head and neck. On moving the head to look down (recall the need for visual reinforcement with tactile/proprioceptive impairment!), both arms will bend up into flexion while both legs brace into extension. When the head is raised to look upwards ('look up while you're walking!') both arms extend and both legs buckle into flexion (that sinking feeling...).

Walking with a Zimmer frame creates obvious difficulties: as the arms brace to take bodyweight for stepping, the legs buckle, and when the legs are braced, the arms buckle (Fig. 5.3). The client's head bobs up and down to alternate the pattern in the struggle for locomotion.

If rehabilitation does not include the re-education of inhibitory processes, the result is an uncontrollable disturbance to – and/or the presentation of – any selective normal movement.

Tonicity

'Muscle tone' refers to the constant state of readiness-to-respond of muscle tissue during waking and resting hours. Normal muscle tone is described as being high enough to sustain a movement against gravity but low enough to allow movement. 'Normal movement' is characterized by the fluency of the grading of muscle tone relative to the force of gravity and the task on hand. It is the primary factor in balance, enabling discrete postural adjustment to give central stability for all mobility.

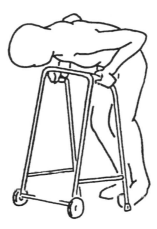

Fig. 5.3 Symmetrical tonic neck reflex in action.

Hypotonicity

Abnormally low tone can be due to disorder in the sensorimotor processing which disturbs the grading of muscle response. It is sometimes confused with the reduced innervation of certain muscles (in whole or in part) caused by focal cell loss in the brain. It can present as a weakness or apparent paralysis of some musculature on the stroke side.

Hypotonicity can also be blamed for what is really a disuse atrophy of the antagonist muscle groups on the stroke side when the stereotypical reflex patterns have become hyperactive. The abdominal muscles are also affected (Davies, 1990). Genuine hypertonicity may impoverish functional movement but seldom interferes with recovering independence including walking, unless cognitive impairments preclude this.

Hypertonicity

Abnormally high tone is due to disorganization in the setting of muscle tonus in the CNS. It presents as undue stiffness or tension in part or all of the body musculature on the stroke-affected side.

The strong antigravity back muscles of the trunk on the stroke side are particularly affected, producing the traditional twisted-backwards posture, hip-hitching and crab-like sidling gait with central instability due to the consequent loss of normal postural adjustments relative to the force of gravity.

Hypertonicity interferes with all natural movement, the ability to move any part of the body fluently. Unchecked, it will also mask and prevent the functional use of recovering movement. In a few cases, usually in more central or brain stem lesions, a general hypertonia can be present. Resembling the rigidity caused by Parkinson's disease, it responds well to small doses of the relevant drugs.

Spasticity

This is a pathological state of ungraded contraction of musculature in response to any stimulus. It does not occur immediately following a stroke unless there is extensive cerebral damage. Usually it is acquired as a result of physiological stressing in the neuromuscular system – plastic reorganization by the accumulative repetition of sustained hypertonicity hyper-reflexia. The presence of spasticity will distort existing normal movement and prevent the re-education of recovering movement. Clinically it presents as:

(1)   Inappropriate co-contraction of muscle groups.
(2)   Non-functional gross movements in reflex patterns in response to stimulation and effort.
(3)   Inability to fractionate these patterns to perform selective movements.
(4)   Increased resistance to passive movement.

Persistent use (physiological stressing) of the non-stroke side in compensatory activity can result in spasticity of this hitherto unaffected side of the body. It can be recognized in a rigidly hunched shoulder ('he has a dropped shoulder on the hemiplegic side'). In effect, he has a raised shoulder on the non-hemiplegic side.

Bobath (1978) observed that weightbearing through the proximal joints (shoulder and hip) on the stroke side appeared to reduce tone in spastic musculature. These areas are now thought to be the site of a secondary segmental system of presynaptic inhibition, and could be the only means of switching on presynaptic inhibitory systems after direct higher CNS control has been lost (Musa, 1986).

Hyper-reflexia

When the sophisticated supraspinal control of inhibition and disinhibition is disrupted, spinal reflex activity is released by the bombardment of sensory stimuli. If these reflex responses are not controlled, the excitability of the response increases with each repetition until even existing or recovering normal movement is pre-empted by the 'hyper-reflexia' of these stereotyped non-purposeful patterns of reflex movement. The plasticity of the neuromuscular system ensures that with this physiological stressing these primitive patterns become self-perpetuating.

Once established, hyper-reflexia is triggered by any effort, either involuntarily as in sneezing, yawning and coughing, or voluntarily by attempting purposeful movement and/or trying too hard to comply with instructions to move.

Recovery from a stroke

The actual effects of a stroke are masked for the first few weeks while the acute inflammation and/or shock response to trauma is resolving. It seems to be during this most vulnerable period, when the fundamental neural repairs are already underway, that the networks influencing the quality of recovery are relaid. The plasticity of the neuromuscular systems ensures that ANY intervention will have a marked effect on the neuromuscular systems – but before rushing headlong to look for miraculous new techniques, it is necessary to determine exactly what we are attempting to rehabilitate.

The relationship between 'recovery' of activity and 'rehabilitation' is more complex than it sounds. The familiar concepts of normal movement in relation to rehabilitation and common-core skills are described in the next chapter – but why does this approach so often fail to produce the results we expect from a seemingly impeccable line of reasoning? Because we need to rebuild the performance of movement, not merely the mechanics of it. The application of any approach depends upon a greater knowledge of this hidden agenda.

The motor control theories discussed here are not divided into Bate's two categories. Clinical insight requires a fuller understanding of all the issues involved, and the suggestion of a dividing line between 'information-processing' and 'action' seems to be unnecessarily restrictive at this stage.

Cognition and motor behaviour

Movements are the output of a dynamic interaction between muscular forces and peripheral field effects such as gravity, friction, and joint reactive forces, and can be described in terms of their pattern, displacement or topology. Movement is the means by which an action is realized. The nature of these means, however, is not fixed or stereotyped but is closely related to the context in which the action takes place. We learn movement by experiencing movement, a process of trial and error to achieve a required goal, as in learning to ride a bicycle.

The classical view on motor control sees the nervous system as a gigantic warehouse of motor engrams of every movement the individual can possibly perform, i.e. the selection of appropriate movements is accomplished by selecting from the warehouse those movement programmes to be activated to fit one's immediate needs.

However, it is now recognized that the traditional concept of 'a motor programme' with retrieval of a complete unit of pre-programmed response cannot explain the infinite flexibility of human motor responses in both novel and familiar actions.

Schmidt (1975, 1976) suggests that the learning of motor skills could be understood in terms of the acquisition of schemata or rules, not as the establishment of specific traces or muscle-specific motor programmes which define only a specific movement sequence, i.e. a constructional view of motor control – that movement representations are not available in ready-made form but have to be constructed according to acquired stored rules (like grammar for language) of 'action schemata'.

He formulated the existence of generalized motor programmes with schemata in relation to perception and visual stimuli. For example, when you see a different breed of dog for the first time, how do you recognize it as a dog? What is stored in the memory cannot be this particular dog but a prototypical abstract knowledge about dogs, and the broadness of this knowledge depends on how many different dogs you have seen in your life.

Relating this to movement: it is possible to write the same phrase with a pen held in the dominant hand, in the dominant hand with the wrist immobilized, in the non-dominant hand, between the toes or gripped between the teeth – and all of these with the paper close to the body, at a distance, and using an assortment of writing materials such as a spraycan, or on sand – spontaneously (albeit perhaps awkwardly) without prior practise. This cannot be explained in terms of units of pre-programmed motor responses.

So, the production of an action may be seen as a generative process in which abstract rules must be transformed into context-specific motor patterns. Galen *et al.* (1990) describe this construction process as involving a multilevel system with higher levels controlling the global aspects of the action such as the functional groupings of muscles constrained to act as a single structure, while the muscle-specific details such as force, velocity and spatial accuracy are considered to be lower-order parametric problems which are dependent on the actual bio-mechanical and environmental context.

Cognitive processes refer to the capacity of the nervous system to store and process environmental information and to use this for the regulation of behaviour. Adams (1981) states that automatized actions are probably per-formed with a minimum cognitive load, whereas novel or complex actions are, for a large part, governed by cognitive mechanisms.

Skilled activities are characterized by more or less automatic and smooth performance, more or less independent of cognitive and perceptual control but still requiring feedback and error-monitoring. Most of our actions such as standing, walking, reaching, are performed without noticeable attention or effort, as are the multitude of actions related to the activities of daily living. They are regulated by means of a mode of control requiring little or no information-processing capacity. Normally this is a fast and fluent process requiring no conscious involvement, but this fluency breaks down after damage to the system. In that case rules are no longer available to control the action (there is 'top-down' disregulation) and peripheral input is no longer able to feed the rules ('bottom-up' disregulation).

Mulder (1991) sees 'impairment' as abnormalities or losses which represent biomechanical disturbances such as muscle strength, range of motion, and sug-gests that 'disabilities' reflect the consequences of impairments in terms of functional performance. Thus analysis of movement refers to the level of impairment only, whereas the analysis of skill refers to the level of disability.

With this interpretation, a disability can be seen as the final result of a breakdown of skill characterized by the non-automatic, jerky performance of a sensorimotor task which becomes largely dependent on cognitive and perceptual guidance, i.e. the loss of sensorimotor adaptability.

An important property of the motor system could be termed 'output constancy', which reflects the tendency of the system to keep the output (action result) constant by continuously adapting the means to the changing internal and/or external conditions. Mulder suggests that the system is able to override control in situations where automaticity is lost, shifting between different modes of control according to the task, the context, and the state of the learner, i.e. when, following a lesion, lower-order (subcortical) control strategies are no longer accessible, the system shifts to higher order (cortical) strategies such as visual or cognitive guidance.

Gaze control

During a discussion on postural control in children with cerebral palsy, Alain Berthoz suggested that the way some of these children roll the head and neck prior to extending neck and head into a relatively stable erect position could be related to the use of vision to replace other impaired afferent signals: the children are visually searching for a high point distally and then by forcing their eyes upwards to this point are able to trigger the required motor action. By being offered a marker such as a bright toy to obtain visual focus, and then raising it slowly, the child is often able to lift the head more directly.

Conversely, when cortical regulation is impoverished, the system relies on lower-order strategies. This is what we are utilizing when we cue or facilitate 'normal' automatic movement responses in our clients. To build schemata for an efficient motor response Mulder suggests that these four factors are stored in memory:

(1) The initial conditions   information about the muscular system and the environment.
(2) The response specifications – speed used, force required, direction of movement and accuracy of the performance.
(3) The sensory consequences – feedback from the sensory systems.
(4) The response outcome – information about the success of the response in relation to the outcome originally intended.

When a number of such movements has been made, an abstract relationship between the four sources develops. The strength of this relation – the schema – determines the flexibility of its usage (c.f. Schmidt's dog analogy).

Biosocial influences

With the physiological and cognitive reprogramming now understood to be taking place in the surviving brain structure following a pathological insult such as a stroke, it is certain that the patterns of emotional response are equally likely to be disrupted and reorganized. Kitwood's (1990, 1997) work is as relevant to neurologically-impaired people of any age as it is to the aged mentally frail (Fig. 5.4).

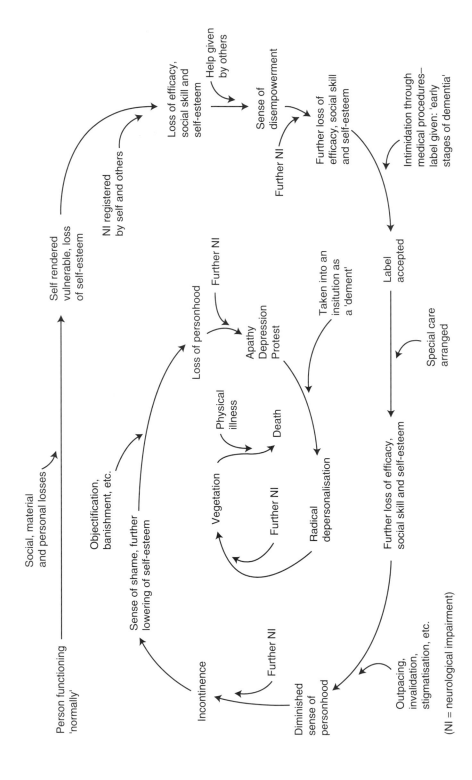

Fig. 5.4   Dialectic on the dementing process (Kitwood, 1990).

In the equation below he places the influence of malignant social psychology (MSP), defined as disempowerment, infantilization, labelling, stigmatization, outpacing, banishment, objectification, etc. (implicated in care models for illness and/or disability)

$$SD = NI + MSP$$

Senile dementia is compounded from the effects of neurological impairment and malignant social psychology.

$$NI <= MSP$$

Neurological impairment attracts a malignant social psychology.

$$MSP => NI$$

Malignant social psychology, bearing down upon a person whose physiological buffers are already fragile, actually creates neurological impairment. This links closely with the evidence on neuromuscular plasticity and the powerful concepts regarding the cognitive control of motor behaviour.

Hickey & Stilwell (1992) state that 'the likelihood that chronic conditions will have negative effects on daily functioning, emphasises the importance of developing treatment strategies consistent with individual needs', and that 'the increasingly recognised importance of the biosocial aspects of disease suggests that healthcare providers may need to spend as much time addressing clients' beliefs and attitudes about illness and its consequences as they do providing clinical treatments'. They go on to note that functional health is now becoming a more useful indicator of health status than medical diagnosis, and that it is also a significant predictor of the use of health and social services.

A study by Partridge *et al.* (1991) found that people's perceptions of their disability varied considerably from that held by the 'professionals'. General levels of independent activity were the factors most highly valued, and the study concluded that intervention should be explicitly related to individually perceived needs. In an earlier study Partridge & Johnson (1989) found that patients with a higher level of control over their recovery actually made more progress.

A joint report by the Royal College of Nursing and the British Geriatric Society in 1975 listed four basic requirements for quality of life:

- Physical (health and functional activity)
- Emotional (loving and being loved)
- Social (fellowship and privacy)
- Psychological (identity and freedom of choice).

In 1992 Gilleard, defining adulthood, listed three essential attributes: identity, autonomy, engagement (social interaction). He maintains that any one of the three can be voluntarily relinquished without loss of adulthood, but that the taking away of any of these elements is an infringement of human rights.

Motivation

Motivation, and the lack of it, has a high profile in medical models of care. Based on purely subjective evidence, this diagnosis is often applied arbitrarily to describe people who are – or who are not – making a 'good' recovery from their stroke. Like everything else to do with this traumatic and complex event, nothing is as simple as it appears.

A good recovery does not depend on good motivation. Only people with a 'mild' stroke (in common parlance, meaning few visible problems) make a good recovery, outwardly, at least. Those with more severe strokes do the best they can with what they have left. Apart from the few clients whose pre-stroke personality influences their adaptation to life post-stroke (some do not have the will to try), the majority of people will desperately wish and work to regain sufficient functional competence to enable an acceptable quality of life. Even those whose cognitive and perceptual deficits preclude active cooperation or full independence will gain considerable improvement from the informed intervention of others.

The reasons for their failure to achieve a predicted outcome can be due to the failure of the rehabilitation process itself to recognize and remediate the cause. Other reasons can include concomitant debilitating pathologies such as chest or urinary infections, constipation, pain (frequently from a traumatized shoulder joint or a chronically sprained ankle), pressure sores (often unnoticed around the stroke ankle), anaemia, malnutrition (swallowing difficulties, inability to reach the cup or cut up the food), cardiac inadequacies, the depletion of stamina and ambition due to the stroke and also the natural ageing processes, and, quite possibly, depression associated with the failure itself.

Depression

Depression is a natural reaction to such a cruelly handicapping condition and will affect enthusiasm and compliance. Altered physicality and the awareness that life will never be the same again, are bitter truths to be absorbed. Clients require unlimited reassurance and understanding and also help with the grieving processes associated with any form of bereavement. Nagging and exhortations to try harder will only increase stress and anxiety (reinforcing spasticity), and add a feeling of guilt, thereby compounding the problem. The prescription of anti-depressant medication will merely cloud the issues and dull the vital 'arousal' level needed to initiate the normal responses to a need to move.

Clinical depression comes later, if at all, unless the client has a known history of depressive illness pre-stroke, and requires expert intervention.

Rehabilitation

The *Community Care Plan 1998–2001*, published by Essex County Council Social Services Department, contains a short statement produced by Essex Disabled People's Association:

> 'The Social Model of Disability relates to how the structure of society and the built environment affects my ability to function and participate in the various aspects of everyday life. It is about the recognition of the need to modify attitudes, and society, by creating awareness of the issues that can lead to an environment that does not disable me.
>
> This is in contrast to the medical model of disability, which implies that I am the problem and need to be cured, modified, or adapted in some way in order to fit into a normal world.'

Taking together the physiological and biosocial aspects, plus all the well-documented evidence that an ability to cope with and enjoy the 'everyday affair' represents the ultimate goal for clients, then maybe we should review the entire rehabilitation process. As Meredith declared in 1991 at a joint conference held by the College of Occupational Therapists and the Chartered Society of Physiotherapy: 'Possibly therapists should be directing their services to solving the problems which are important to their clients, and not assuming that they understand or know what is best.'

Re-learning motor behaviour

Rosenbaum (1991) and Mulder & Gunts (1993) have demonstrated that goals can be reached by means of numerous movement combinations and that an identical combination is almost never repeated. The behavioural output is continuously being changed in response to internal and external cues. Even in the spinal cord, pools of motor neuron activity are constantly being shifted around, so that output patterns are never exactly the same.

Schmidt (1976) concludes that motor skills are learned by the acquisition of schemata or rules. As in his examples of dog recognition and *ad hoc* writing, a rich experience is required to develop an outline. Neurorehabilitation therefore can only be effective if these schemata are replaced, or rebuilt if destroyed or rendered inaccessible by the lesion.

Mulder lists four factors which are fundamental to the re-acquisition of a schema:

(1)   Variability of practice.
(2)   Consistent use of feedback.
(3)   Relationship between the therapy and activities of daily living.
(4)   Emphasis on achievements instead of passive guidance.

Variability of practice

If during motor learning and re-learning we are acquiring action schemata, this implies that learning by means of the repetition of isolated non-action-specific movement will be useless. If therapy is developing the acquisition of schemata or prototypical knowledge about the skill under training, then it follows that the quality of the required schema depends largely on the variability of practice. Taken in conjunction with the plasticity of the neuromuscular system, only the faithful repetition of normal movement patterns in all relevant situations will rehabilitate sensorimotor skills effectively.

Consistent use of feedback

Normally all our movements are accompanied by a continuous stream of afferent information for monitoring performance and correcting errors. After CNS trauma, the resulting impairment may offer incomplete or distorted afferent data, and/or the feedback loops can themselves be disturbed or disregulated.

If Response Outcome is one of the four sources of information essential to the development of action schemata then, without appropriate feedback, errors cannot be noted and improvement cannot occur. To be effective, therapy has to generate the relevant feedback information, including both verbal commentary and physical demonstration.

Carrol & Bandura (1982, 1985), Whiting *et al.* (1987) have shown that observational learning is extremely relevant for the acquisition of motor skills, but the use of video and 'live' modelling remains surprisingly under-used in working practice.

However, use of this supplementary sensory feedback has to be vigorously monitored itself, continuously assessed and sensitively withdrawn to enable any restoration of self-sufficient sensorimotor adaptability to take place. Neuro-rehabilitation utilizes the full range of sensory stimulation for feedback and feedforward – cortical and subcortical clueing, cueing, and facilitation – to prompt normal movement responses, but appropriate weaning from dependency on our input is a vital factor in the recovery process.

Therapy and activities of daily living

Carr & Shepherd (1989), like Bobath, from a rich background of clinical experience, associate motor relearning with the use of familiar and task-specific activity. When this is related to the rest of the evidence, and the concept that actual motor learning is of goal-directed actions rather than of muscle-specific combinations, then we have to accept that a therapy focused at the level of muscles and joint movements – aimed at restoring distorted elements instead of distorted actions – will result in the development of a very narrow schema indeed which is of no practical value in everyday living.

To strengthen the value of a schema for regaining functional activity, therapy needs to be structured in such a way that practise takes place in a widely variable context (extending to leisure activities also), with maximum overlap between the therapeutic situation and the ordinary daily life situation. If there is a large gap between these situations, then the scheme acquired during therapy will be of no use for the activities of daily living.

The problem with 'carry-over' implies that all rehabilitationists need to rebuild the 'grammar' of movement first in order to reinforce or replace the cognitive scaffolding.

Active movements vs passive guidance

Although many rehabilitation techniques involve some form of guidance through the task on hand, this only affects the mechanical condition of the musculo-skeletal system. It eliminates the learner's need to select the appropriate response: it does not result in motor learning (Mulder, 1992).

In neuromuscular terms, dynamic movement is significantly related to the neurophysiological factors involved in the control of muscle tonus and reflex activity. Remember that basic movement patterns generated from spinal cord programmes (reflex activity) are initiated and modified by input from both the CNS and the periphery (appearing to come from the proximal regions of the limbs, the receptors so far unidentified). In 1978 Bobath found that movement or change in position of proximal limb joints can both reduce spasticity and reflex activity and facilitate normal movement.

Musa (1991) suggests that following CNS damage, this secondary system of pre-synaptic inhibition may be the only way to switch on the higher pre-synaptic inhibitory mechanisms. Restoration of postural control against gravity also requires dynamic activity to stimulate feedback/feedforward systems. Carr & Shepherd (1989) summarize three major findings from other research programmes which show that postural adjustments are:

(1) Anticipatory and ongoing: for example preparatory adjustments ensure that the potentially de-stabilizing effect of an arm movement is countered before it occurs.
(2) Task- and context-specific: muscle activation patterns vary according to the position of the individual, the task being performed, and the context in which it occurs.
(3) Visually affected: vision provides critical information about body position in space which is of course directly relevant to the anticipatory factor. Without sophisticated postural control against gravity giving central stability, no functional limb movements are possible.

Static postures in themselves contribute to many more problems than pressure sores, boredom, and impoverished stimulation for cognitive motor relearning and neurophysiological restructuring. Immobilization and lack of use can, moreover, lead to atrophy. Neurodynamics indicates that: 'adverse neural tension', the biomechanical stressing of nerve tissue, will compound the problems of stroke. Butler (1991) warns that sitting in the 'slump' position actually lengthens the spinal cord and peripheral nerves by some 5–8cms and pulls on the brain stem structure. After only 15% elongation, the walls of the feeder arteries are so narrowed that adequate circulation is seriously restricted, leading to degeneration of neural and intraneural tissues. This affects the innervation of afferent and efferent pathways, creating further problems with motor behaviour and activity.

Many stroke survivors spend a considerable time slump-sitting in wheelchairs, dayrooms or beside their beds. This also creates changes in both the visual and vestibular concept of space and posture, so that even previously unimpaired normal posture and postural adjustments are re-adjusted to make standing erect and balancing even more difficult.

Rehabilitation outcomes

Conventionally, outcome is measured in terms of the visible motor output in isolation: can he walk, how far and how fast, make a cup of tea, communicate basic needs'. But how many stroke survivors appear to achieve measurable results in the formal therapy environment without regaining any actual coping skills in social and domestic settings or confidence in their abilities, or quality of life?

If we accept that motor, sensory and cognitive factors interact seamlessly in the re-acquisition of motor behaviour, then all of these factors should be part of any assessment procedure focused on the recovery of an acceptable standard of habilitation.

In 1995 Mulder *et al.* outlined three stages in motor learning (c.f. learning to ride a bicycle):

(1) The cognitive stage in which the learner makes an initial approximation to the skill based on background (tacit) knowledge, observation and instruction.
(2) The associative stage in which the performance is refined through the elimination of errors.
(3) The autonomous stage in which skilled performance is well-established.

The principles of functional reorganization can be distilled from the work undertaken in recent years in Njimegen, that functional recovery is reflected by:

- A decrease in cognitive regulation.
- A decrease in visual dependency.

- A restoration of sensorimotor adaptability (the fast and fluent multilevel (cortical/subcortical) processing of information necessary for any skilled performance).

It follows that shifts in the re-acquisition of this motor learning, re-learning and control, across time, give an objective indication of recovery.

Mulder has suggested that these signs of recovery have more relevance for the prediction of performance in daily life activities than the conventional bio-mechanical parameters, and could provide an objective tool for both clinical measurement and predictive assessment.

The clinical imperative

This chapter has reviewed the compelling evidence which shows why a colla-borative approach is needed; it also offers credible explanations for the poor results achieved even from some intensive rehabilitation procedures and pro-vides a firmer foundation for clinical reasoning in neurorehabilitation. This evidence should be incorporated into every model of stroke management.

No standardized routine of exercises or techniques can ever be effective for all stroke-impaired clients. Each individual presents a different range of problems, similar sometimes but never the same. As adults we have all developed a very personal neuromuscular system with programmed behavioural codes relevant to our own social and environmental requirements.

Neuromuscular plasticity

Physiological stressing, by habitual patterns of movement, forms networks for the automatic reproduction of these movements and hardwires in good and bad patterns indiscriminately, from the moment of trauma onwards. Inconsistent use of existing, recovering and re-educated activity wrecks progress by failing to reinforce normal performance in a time of CNS confusion. Practise makes per-fect, imperfect practise makes imperfect. Abnormal motor patterns comprising uninhibited reflex activity and the resultant spasticity, non-use of hemiplegic limbs, over-compensatory movement, unnecessary dependency on physical assistance from others – these are secondary disabilities acquired after the stroke as a result of uninformed management.

Regarding the cognitive control of motor behaviour: working on the mechanical components of a movement or skill does not rehabilitate perfor-mance. Skilled performance requires the re-acquisition of schemata by facil-itating 'normal' movement patterns in familiar task and context-specific situations in a broad range of everyday environments. To assist this process occupational therapists, physiotherapists and nurses need to relax certain pro-fessional boundaries regarding core expertise and to share common-core skills.

In addition assessment procedures need to be revised to reflect the more realistic aspects of recovery. The patterns of recovery and final outcome are unpredictable, and specialized intervention is not always available. From the moment of the stroke onwards the priorities for everyone must be to:

(1) Prevent the acquisition of secondary disabilities.
(2) Guide forward the recovering functional ability.
(3) Ensure the ongoing use of functional ability.
(4) Reinforce progress.

The biosocial aspects of recovery involve many people and considerable 'hands-on' intervention. Helping someone who is unable to fend for themselves can border closely upon invasion of privacy and infringement of human rights. The 'medical model' of healthcare deprives most people with long-term disabilities of their autonomy, their identity, and their recognized place in the family and in society. The recipients are at risk of losing dignity. The traditional system of rehabilitation reinforces the loss. One of our responsibilities to each individual should be the restoration of a sense of personal autonomy, of regaining control and personal responsibility, of coping without us, so that discharge from The System does not leave clients still clinging to the wreckage of their former selves.

A stroke-impaired client is in a neurologically critical condition, totally susceptible to neurological and cognitive reorganization. In all activity, from the initial approach at every contact to active intervention, we are manipulating mature brain activity – we are engaged in trophic engineering. The responsibility for the outcome is entirely ours – by updating our clinical reasoning, we have in place a framework for effective rehabilitation.

References

Adams, J.A. (1981) Do cognitive factors in motor performance become non-functional with practice? *Journal of Motor Behaviour* **13**, 262–73.

Bach-y-Rita, P. (1981) Central nervous system lesions: sprouting and unmasking in rehabilitation. *Archives of Phys Med Rehabilitation* **62**, 413–17.

Bate, P. (1997) Motor control theories: insights for therapists. *Physiotherapy* **83**, 397–405.

Bishop, B. (1982) Neural plasticity. *Physical Therapy* **62**(8), 1132–82 and **62**(9), 1275–82.

Bisiach, E. & Luzzatti, C. (1978) Unilateral Neglect of Representational Space Cortex **14**, 129–33.

Bobath, B. (1978) Personal communication.

Bobath, B. (1963) Treatment principles and planning in cerebral palsy. *Physiotherapy* **49**, 122–4.

Bobath, B. (1990) *Adult Hemiplegia: Evaluation and Treatment*, 3rd edn. Heinemann, London.

Brown, M.A. & Hardman, V.J. (1987) Plasticity of Vertebrate Mononeurons. In *Growth and Plasticity of Neural Connections* (W. Winslow & C. McCrohan, eds), pp. 36–51. Manchester University Press, Manchester.

Butler, D. (1991) *Mobilisation of the Nervous System.* Churchill Livingstone, London.

Carr, J.H. & Shepherd, R.B. (1989) A motor learning model for stroke rehabilitation. *Physiotherapy* **75**(7), 372–80.

Carrol, W.R. & Bandura, A. (1982) The role of visual monitoring in observational learning of action patterns. *Journal of Motor Behaviour* **14**, 153–67.

Carrol, W.R. & Bandura, A. (1985) The role of timing of visual monitoring and motor rehearsal on observational learning of action patterns. *Journal of Motor Behaviour* **17**, 269–83.

Davies, P. (1990) *Right in the Middle: Selective Trunk Activity.* Springer-Verlag, Berlin.

Epstein, W. (1986) Contrasting conceptions of perception and action. *Acta Psychologica* **63**, 103–15.

van Galen, G.P., Van Doorn, R.R.A. & Schmaaker, L.R.B. (1990) Effects of motor programming on power spectral density function of finger and wrist movements. *Journal of Exptl Psychology* **16**, 755–65.

Gilleard, C.J. (1992) Losing one's mind and losing one's place; a psychosocial model of dementia. In *Gerontology: Responding to an Ageing Society* (K. Morgan, ed.), pp. 149–56. Jessica Kingsley, London.

Hickey, T. & Stillwell, D.L. (1992) Chronic illness and ageing: a personal-contextual model of age-related changes in health status. *Gerontology* **18**, 1–15.

Hertanu, J.S., Demopoulos, J.T., Yang, W.C., Calhoun, W.F. & Fenigstein, H.A. (1984) Stroke rehabilitation: correlation and prognostic value of computerised tomography and sequential functional assessments. *Archives of Phys Med Rehab* **65**, 505.

Humphreys & Riddoch (1987)

Kidd, G., Lawes, N. & Musa, I.M. (1992) *Understanding Neuromuscular Plasticity: A Basis for Clinical Rehabilitation.* Edward Arnold, London.

Kitwood, T. (1990) The dialectics of dementia: with particular reference to Alzheimer's disease. *Ageing and Society* **10**(2), 177–96.

Kittwood, T. (1997) *Dementia Revisited.* Open University Press, Milton Keynes.

Klein, M.R. (1976) Attention and movement. In *Motor Control: Issues and Trends* (G.E. Stelmach, ed.). Academic Press, New York.

Laidler, P. (1994) *Stroke Rehabilitation: Structure and Strategy.* Chapman & Hall, London/Stanley Thornes, Cheltenham.

Mulder, Th. (1991) A process-oriented model of human motor behaviour: towards a theory-based rehabilitation approach. *Physical Therapy* **71**(2), 157–64.

Mulder, Th. (1992) Current ideas on motor control and learning: implications for therapy. In *Spinal Cord Dysfunction 2 – Intervention and Treatment* (L.S. Illis, ed.). Oxford University Press, Oxford.

Mulder, Th. & Gunts, A.C.H. (1993a) Recovery of motor skill following nervous system disorder: a behavioural emphasis. In *Bailliere's Clinical Neurology* **2**, pp. 1–13.

Mulder, Th. (1993b) Learning Motor Skills. In *Proceedings of the 3rd Symposium of the Graduate Institute of Human Movement* (C.A.M. Doorenbosch *et al.*, eds). Free University Press, Amsterdam.

Mulder, Th., Pauwels, J. & Mienhuis, B. (1995) Motor recovery following stroke: towards a disability-orientated assessment of motor dysfunction. In *Physiatry in Stroke Management* (M.A. Harrison, ed.).

Musa, I.M. (1986) The role of afferent input in the reduction of spasticity: an hypothesis. *Physiotherapy* **72**(4), 179–81.

Musa, I.M. (1991) The role of afferent input in the reduction of spasticity: an hypothesis. *Physiotherapy* **72**(4), 179–82.

Partridge, C.J. & Johnson, M. (1989) Perceived control of recovery from physical disability: measurement and prediction. *British Journal of Psychology* **28**, 53–9.

Partridge, G.J. *et al.* (1991)

Rawlings, C., Rossitch, E. & Nashold, B.F. The history of neurosurgical procedures for the relief of pain. *Surgical Neurology* **38**, 454–63.

Reber, A.S. (1989) Implicit learning and tacit knowledge. *Journal of Experimental Psychology* **118**, 219–35.

Rosenbaum, D.A. (1991) *Human Motor Control.* Academic Press, New York.

Schmidt, R.A. (1975) A schema theory of discrete motor learning. *Psychological Review* **82**, 225–60.

Schmidt, R.A. (1976) The schema as a solution to some persistent problems in motor learning theory. In *Motor Control: Issues and Trends* (G.E. Stelmach, ed.). Academic Press, New York.

Whiting, H.T.A., Bijlard, M.J. & den Brinker, B. (1987) The effect of the availability of a dynamic model on the acquisition of a complex cyclical action. *Quarterly Journal of Exptl Psychology* **39a**, 153–67.

Wise, S.P. & Desimone, R. (1988) Behavioural neuropsychology: insights into seeing and grasping. *Science* **242**, 736–40.

Chapter 6
Rehabilitating Movement
Polly Laidler

Rehabilitation for stroke survivors requires multidisciplinary input. No single profession can accommodate the depth of knowledge nor the range of expertise needed to identify and remediate all the complex problems resulting from the stroke. Moreover, because of the quality and quantity of neuroscientific discrimination involved, stroke rehabilitation is a specialized field for each profession.

However, the periods of specialized input are limited even in designated stroke units, and usually taper away completely soon after discharge into the community. For most of the time professional colleagues and others are working with and caring for the stroke-disabled, and it is the quality and quantity of this continuous input/output control that is the major influence on their progress. In the hospital environment the nursing teams, and elsewhere significant others such as carers, spouses, partners, are in truth the primary, front-line, rehabilitationists.

This influential stressing of normal performance in all the activities of daily living and the prevention of all the secondary disabilities, 24 hours a day, requires merely an awareness of normal movement relative to gravity, the sharing of identified common-core skills and generous interdisciplinary communication. Without this simple background of informed practice, despite rigorous sessions with specialized therapists, the majority of stroke survivors will be unable to achieve their potential to return to a relatively normal lifestyle.

Physiotherapy core expertise includes the re-education and rehabilitation of movement. Movement however is an integral component in almost all activity and, of course, is involved in the rehabilitation of any disability by any discipline in any setting (the posture and performance of clients in arriving, in taking off/putting on clothing, sitting, turning, using tools such as pen/paper, in eating and drinking, getting up, departing). Therefore a knowledge of 'normal' movement and its importance should underpin all input and be passed on to all staff and domestic carers appropriately.

To avoid undue repetition, the side of the body affected by the stroke is designated the 'stroke' side and written as S (S arm, S leg, etc). The 'non-stroke-affected' side is written as N (N arm), and 'left' as L and 'right' as R. For simplicity the term 'helper' is used indiscriminately – it could be a therapist, a nurse, an aide or assistant, a porter, professionally qualified persons or a domestic carer.

This chapter gives guidelines to the facilitation and control of movement and examines their application to everyday activities (the relevance of familiar task-specific activity to stroke rehabilitation is validated in Chapter 5). General principles and common-core skills are worked through stage-by-stage first, followed by a review of some physiotherapy strategies in a departmental setting.

The definition if iatrogenesis is appropriate here: 'Any adverse mental or physical condition induced in a patient by the effects of treatment by a physician or surgeon (Taber's *Cyclopedic Medical Dictionary*) – or by a therapist, a nurse, or any member of staff...'. The definition also implies that such effects could have been avoided by proper and judicious care on the part of the practitioner (El-Din, 1991) such as sharing information with family carers and includes sins of omission (Laidler, 1994).

Therefore, some traditional but dangerously outdated doctrines are also included as 'lame dogmas' with appropriate clarification.

General principles

Normal movement

This is the acquired co-ordinated purposeful, fluent, skilful and appropriate use of body and limbs in relation to the earth's gravitational field. The baseline for all movement is postural control against gravity. This is acquired from birth onwards, through a process of trial and error for all new activity until a successful outcome is achieved (the winning formulae of action schemata or programming rules to initiate context-specific motor actions are then 'on file' for use in all contextual situations). This postural adaptability enables selective movement.

Balance

The primary aim of physical neurorehabilitation is to restore dynamic postural stability. The centre of gravity (CoG) in adult humans can be imagined as being mid-chest (over-simplistic, but adequate for this purpose), around the lower section of the sternum and halfway between front and back.

What holds us up from the ground can be called the base of support (BoS). In standing, this is the length of our feet and the width between them. In sitting the BoS is larger – from toe-tip to back of buttocks (or rump); and if leaning back into a chair the BoS extends to where the shoulders, neck or head touch the chairback. Lying prone or supine offers the maximum area of support. Obviously the larger the BoS, the safer we feel: sitting feels safer than standing, standing on one leg is far less secure than standing on two. The smaller the BoS, the greater the demand on the postural musculature, both in effort and in co-ordinated tone-graded interplay, to hold the body in position against the force of gravity.

The CoG over the BoS in any position gives stability. When it falls outside the BoS, we are 'off-balance' and fall down unless we can utilise all the counter-balancing head, trunk and limb movements to regain stability.

Moving the CoG in relation to the BoS gives mobility with stability and brings in all the balance and 'righting' reactions painstakingly acquired since birth. 'Facilitation of normal movement patterns' utilizes this factor.

Stroke-impaired movement

A stroke disrupts the sophisticated neuromuscular postural adjustments to gravity. In most cases the S side of the trunk musculature becomes hypertonic and subject to uninhibited reflexes, as are the S limbs. All the balance and righting reactions are affected: every movement of an arm or a leg becomes harder and more hazardous or even impossible without this background of anticipatory, immediate and ongoing postural adaptation to the changing distribution of weight. The effect is more noticeable of course as the BoS is reduced: coming up to stand from a sitting position, activities in standing, and walking, are the most demanding.

Without the vital background of fluent postural adjustment to sustain central stability, selective functional limb movement cannot be performed 'normally'. Humans have to resort to quadrupedal propping, using the arm(s) as an extra leg to hold a rigid trunk against gravity. Hands are no longer sophisticated tools in their own right but are used as safety props on furniture or walking aid; letting go even to turn a door handle can be difficult and risky, at times impossible.

All rehabilitation therefore is concentrated throughout on restoring, re-educating and reinforcing automatic postural adjustment to gravity to enable the stroke survivor to use recovering abilities.

Normal sensorimotor adaptability

The appropriate ranging between cognitive cortical (higher) and subcortical (lower) systems is highly energy efficient. Little of our energy potential is consumed by routine or familiar tasks because they are dealt with by the acquired 'automatic' responses. The rest is held in reserve to be utilized as required for the acquisition of new skills, processing new information, dealing with new situations, etc. This accounts for the high level of fatigue experienced by stroke survivors – every movement needed to perform a task (including postural adjustments) has to be concentrated on and performed 'consciously'.

Frequent rest periods are necessary particularly in the early months, as energy reserves are exhausted very quickly and are being continuously depleted by ongoing activity until sufficient sensorimotor adaptability is re-established to enable some return to more normal performance levels. As this is likely to remain impoverished, many people who have had a stroke may suffer always from reduced stamina.

Following a stroke, even if it is classed as a 'minor' event, fluency of movement and the ability to dance, run, jump, swim, play a musical instrument requiring ambidexterity, usually remains impaired. People will never feel the same as they did before, as there is always some residual handicap, maybe not always visible to a casual observer (frequently this is an even more disabling cognitive or perceptual loss).

Give plenty of hope and confidence in ongoing improvement but do not give unattainable goals by over-emphasis on a regime which seems to promise the positive restoration of 'normal movement' in all activity; stroke survivors eagerly leap to erroneous conclusions. The relentless striving for perfection is the therapist's hidden agenda, and should not be downloaded on to a vulnerable client! Help the individual and the family to come to terms with the situation from the beginning: enable a realistic but philosophical adjustment to an arbitrary change in fortune and encourage enjoyment in life after a stroke, whatever the consequences of it may be.

'The important thing is to add life to years, not years to life' (Amulree).

Common core skills

The appropriate and consistent handling and positioning of stroke-impaired clients, and the use of strategies such as 'facilitation' and 'subcortical stimulation', ensures that physiological and cognitive stressing will enable clients to reach their optimum potential recovery.

This principle applies to everyone working with and caring for a stroke survivor in all the activities of daily living. Moving in bed, washing, dressing, getting on and off the lavatory or commode, eating, participating in leisure activities, getting to and from the therapy sessions – all involve movement which has to be moulded or remodelled into more 'normal' patterns for ongoing recovery, at all times, for as long as it takes (or as far as possible). The carefully structured, supervized and monitored performance of all daily (and nightly) activity is vital to the successful outcome of any rehabilitation programme. Remember, without collaboration no specialized 'therapy' sessions can be effective. Everybody has to be involved in the process and made more aware of the nature of movement that most of us take for granted.

Start by observing how other, unimpaired, people move; watch for the subtle changes in position prior to any actual activity, and think too about your own abilities. Notice the easy turns at wrist and elbow, slight stretch forward of shoulder region and the changing angles of fingers and thumb when picking up a mug of tea, for example. During the next trip to the loo, test the subtle acrobatics – involving all limbs as well as head, neck and trunk – required in reaching for toilet paper and using it. And try using your other hand to cope in these situations.

Handling

The amount of assistance needed by stroke-disabled people has to be carefully adjusted to each individual, to fill in the obvious gaps in their capability, so that the recipient is still able to participate and feel in control of the move, the movement, and the action, wherever possible. Total help (lifting, washing/dressing) is seldom justified except in certain very early or severe cases, and even here active awareness and participation must be encouraged. When someone is totally dependent upon a nurse or carer, the stroke-affected limbs and the position of head and trunk need to be moved in just the same way that they would be moving and re-adjusting into place independently, with body and limbs co-ordinating together to come to rest in another position.

Lame dogmas:
● 'It's quicker to do it for them'.
● 'It won't matter just for once'.

It isn't quicker, in the long run, as the person will progress rapidly to requiring little or no help. And it will matter, as 'just once' is seldom just once, and even once unravels and replaces the recovery underway; it disables people.

Handling hazards

The shoulder   The 'shoulder' is comprised of several joints making up the shoulder girdle. The scapula is embedded in the posterior muscles of the trunk which are usually abnormally high-toned after a stroke: this prevents the normal sliding action that enables all arm movement. The glenohumeral joint, where the arm anchors into the shoulder girdle, is formed by a small vertical 'saucer' on the scapula into which the head of the humerus nestles. It is held in place by a cartilaginous cuff strengthened by tendinous ligaments and by support from the muscles over and around it (the deltoid taking most of the weight of the arm against the force of gravity). The effective activity of these muscles will be depleted on the stroke side, so the weight of an unsupported arm is taken by the thin inelastic cuff which alone cannot hold the joint aligned against gravity.

Lame dogmas:
● 'Maintain full range of movement (RoM) in the S shoulder joint to prevent adhesions.'
● 'A painful shoulder is just another syndrome associated with stroke.'

Both these statements are dangerously wrong. Unless there is full and free and normal reciprocal movement in the entire shoulder-girdle mechanism (which is extremely unlikely), ANY movement of the S arm whether assisted by others, used to pull or lift someone into position, or enthusiastically performed by the stroke survivor using the N hand to haul it about, will result in trauma by:

- tearing the connective tissue structures around the gleno-humeral joint;
- possibly rupturing the cuff allowing the head of the humerus to dislocate (usually ending up wedged anteriorly under the clavicle);
- eventually wrenching the scapula from the hypertonic back muscles.

The traditional 'painful shoulder' is usually a result of inflicted or self-inflicted injury, however well-intentioned to begin with; this is iatrogenic. It may also be the final outcome of uninhibited hyper-reflexive activity in the muscles acting on the glenohumeral joint. The 'waiter's tip' reflex pulls the arm down, into medial (inward) rotation, and across the front of the chest (feel the tension in the pectoral muscles on the S side) aided by the flexor-pattern reflexes.

The hypertonic trunk musculature on the S side reinforced by extensor-patterned reflexia is pulling the arm also into medial rotation, downwards and backwards. The head of the humerus is therefore subjected to violent forces predominantly twisting it out of the 'socket' and into anterior wedging again under the clavicle. It is iatrogenic to allow this to happen: reflex activity and hypertonic trunk musculature can and should be controlled.

The ankle   The ankle joint is also composed of more than one joint, held together by the capsules and stronger ligaments, and by the tendon insertions of muscles into and over the joints. Abnormal reflex activity twists the foot inwards into inversion, the extensor pattern adds plantarflexion; any weightbearing over the foot in these positions will 'sprain' the ankle, tearing/rupturing some or all the protective tissues. Acute trauma brings oedema and inflammation; persistent trauma produces permanent damage.

It is iatrogenic. Always check that the S foot is positioned correctly, flat on the floor, before attempting to move a client or allowing them to move themselves.

Positioning and moving

From the moment of admission (or the stroke itself if the individual is not hospitalised) everything and everybody around the client should be working to ensure that the client is utilizing the secondary systems of presynaptic inhibition located in the proximal joints of the body, the shoulders and hips ('weightbearing on the affected side') in order to prevent the establishing of stereotyped reflexes leading to spasticity.

Furniture (bed, bedside locker, chair/s) needs to be placed so that most activity takes place on the S side. This will direct attention to this side and encourage head-turning and instinctive transference of bodyweight to this side. It is doubly important if there is perceptual 'unilateral neglect'. In these cases, start with objects and people set to the front and encourage eye contact, then move the set gradually (may take a day or two) to the S side to introduce scanning and attention into the 'missing' areas of extrapersonal space.

Lame dogma:
- Some practitioners still advocate dealing totally to the N side 'for the patient's convenience', but this will of course only reinforce the problems. It is iatrogenic (see Figs 6.1, 6.2 and 6.3 below).

For resting positions, ensure regular distribution of bodyweight through the S shoulder and hip. Assistance should always be offered to and from the S side: this also blocks any tendency to fall to this side or to roll too close to the edge of the bed.

Lying down positions

On the S side: the S shoulder has to be positioned well forwards so that bodyweight is taken through the scapula and not directly on to the point of the shoulder itself. Lying on the S side means that the N arm is free to reach for things, this naturally rolls a little more weight over the S side each time. The underneath (S) leg needs to be fairly straight at the hip.

On the N side: the S shoulder is placed comfortably forwards with the arm and hand supported. Lying on one's back is not recommended – the S limbs fall into the reflex patterns (arm flexed and held into the chest, leg resting in lateral (outward) rotation with knee extended and foot planarflexed (pointing down) and inverting (turning in) at the ankle), and all the bony pressure areas are at risk.

Sitting in a chair

Some bodyweight should be relayed up into the S shoulder via the S elbow and forearm. Ensure that the S arm is positioned forward so that the shoulder joint is correctly aligned, and the S wrist and hand are supported. If a table is unavailable, then use cushions/pillows on the lap, or the wide arm of an armchair. In the early stages it is advisable to have a thin cushion, towel or drawsheet under the client – it makes assisted re-positioning much easier.

The rump should sit firmly against the back of the chair, backside level. With heightened tone in the back muscles on the S side, the trunk will be pulled further back at that side. It will also twist the trunk to the S side, raising the buttock, so that bodyweight is shifted towards the N side and off the S hip. If this is happening, the N hip needs to be further back to bring the S hip slightly forwards. Bodyweight must be evenly distributed through both hips. Check hip levels from behind the client, and help to adjust bodyweight over the S side if necessary with a quick lift-and-tug upwards from the N side of the pelvis (trouser waistbands are ideal for the purpose) to roll the weight across. If sitting on a cushion/towel/cloth, then this can be lugged upwards on the S side instead.

Feet should be flat on the floor, heels well down particularly on the S foot (see Fig. 6.4).

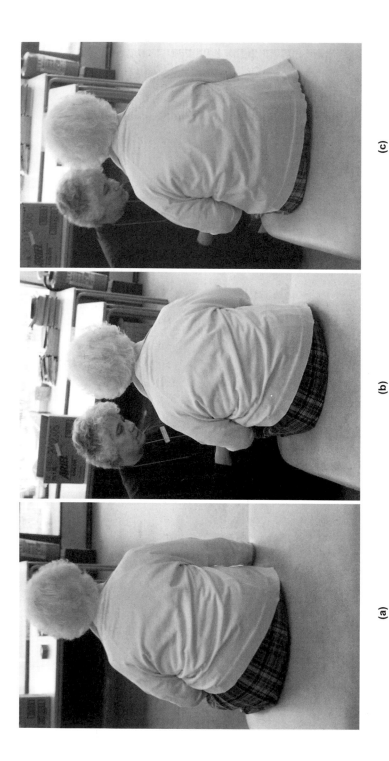

(a)

(b)

(c)

Fig. 6.1 (a) Sitting posture needs to be recognized and adjusted before any further movement takes place.
(b) A little firm downward pressure is offered to the S knee to ensure a positive bracing response as the proximal keypoint is used to stimulate a normal sitting to standing movement. Then 'hands-off' to allow natural sway and balance reactions, while being ready to support if needed.
(c) Progress to facilitating sitting-to-standing from the central keypoint only, by controlling the centre of gravity forwards and upwards over the base of support during the activity until the patient has regained the postural stability to manage this for herself. The patient displays the potential to achieve independent transfers, stepping and walking if given effective follow-through from the staff at the residential care home.

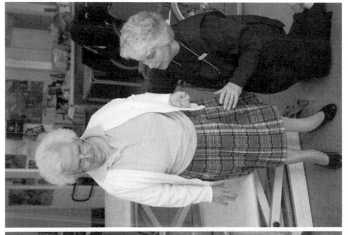

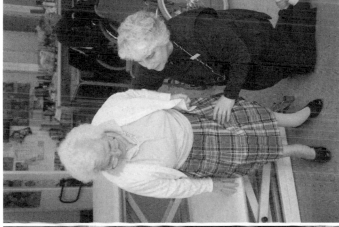

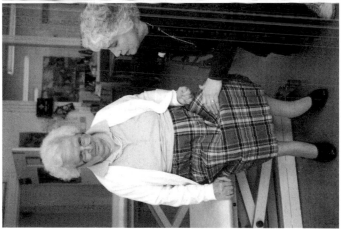

Fig. 6.2 Sitting to standing.

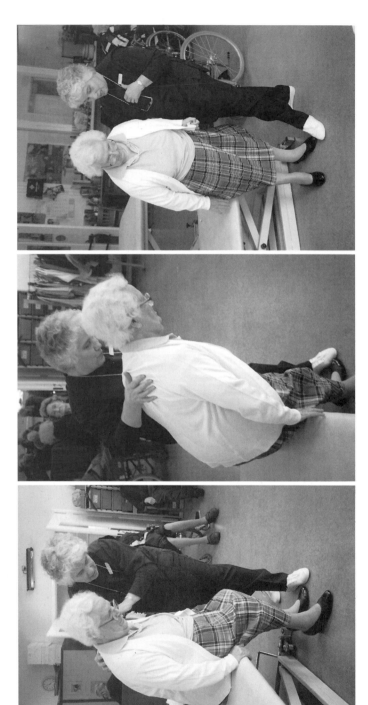

Fig. 6.3   Getting up to the S side is not only easier than to the N side but it may also stimulate some normal response from the S arm. Assistance is given only where necessary to prevent undue effort.

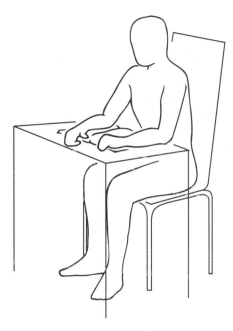

Fig. 6.4 Correct sitting position in a chair.

Moving techniques

Turning and rolling Always encourage the stroke-disabled person to look and feel to both sides (using the N arm/hand only, if the S one can't) to ensure that there is sufficient space for the manoeuvre. This helps re-orientation and spatial awareness.

To the N side: assistance may be needed to bring the S shoulder and arm forwards to start the roll – guiding from over the scapula area with great care (not by pulling on the S arm).

To the S side: bring the N arm over the body to 'reach' across, forwards and downwards, to rest the hand on the S side of the bed (reassuring to the client, who can then control any tendency to go on rolling off), and assist with a hand behind the N shoulder if necessary to initiate the roll-over. The legs will naturally follow.

Sitting up on the side of the bed Getting up to the S side is not only easier than to the N side but may also stimulate some normal response from the S arm. The N arm can push up from the side of the bed which is a good start towards independent activity (otherwise it has to pull on something or someone), bodyweight is rolled over the S hip which inhibits unwanted reflex activity, and normal balance reactions are stimulated as the head and trunk come upright. As the body rights itself, both legs with knees bent can swing forward over the edge of the bed.

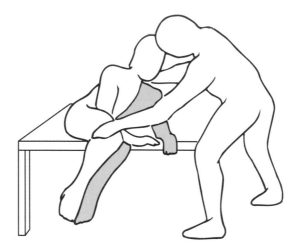

Fig. 6.5a Rolling over to sit on the side of the bed.

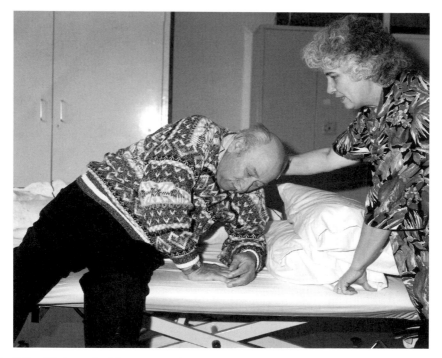

Fig. 6.5b Photograph of the movement.

Assistance is given as necessary (avoid struggle, as this stimulates reflexes) by giving support with one hand behind the S shoulder and the other under the client's knees to guide the follow-through.

It is important to get people accustomed to getting out of bed to their S side, to gain maximum dynamic activity over the S side of the body. Use 'hip-hitching' (described below) to bring a client nearer to the edge of the bed prior to another manoeuvre.

Swivel transfer between the two seats (maximum assistance)   Surfaces should, ideally, be at a right angle to each other and about the same height. Test the manoeuvre several times for yourself and then with a colleague as 'helper'. When working with a colleague, notice that you need plenty of space to avoid head-butting, so give the client sufficient space by standing well to the S side.

Without using your hands to push up, swing your rump up and over into the second chair WITHOUT standing up or taking a step. Feet should swivel appropriately if they start apart with heels angled towards the right-angle. Straightening up necessitates taking little steps in order to back into the new position in front of the second chair. Allowing someone to actually stand up with straightened knees instantly raises the CoG and puts the body into an unstable start. Stepping involves taking one foot off the floor which is even worse.

Facilitate 'hip-hitching' the client's rump nearer to the front of the seat, if necessary by grasping and gently rocking the pelvis from side to-side: as the bodyweight is rolled on to one buttock, the other side plus thigh can be lifted forwards (or use the cushion/towel, grasped at each side). This simple procedure, introduced at this very early stage and practised until the client can do it inde pendently, helps to re-educate postural control for the crucial transference of weight (the genuine shift-over balance to lift one leg up, a much reduced BoS) for standing and stepping and walking.

Feet should be positioned roughly halfway between the two seats to avoid the need to take a step. Clients should hold their hands linked together (no need to interlink fingers) using the self-help hold for the S hand and wrist (S wrist cradled in N hand, N thumb exerting pressure into the S palm up to the fingers, to maintain extension in the S wrist). This overcomes the temptation to clutch at helper or furniture during the move.

If physically frail in other ways (arthritis, very old age) then a push up from the bed or the arm of the chair, using both hands if possible – otherwise, just the N hand, followed by a reach across to support on the arm of the second chair, is quite permissible!

The helper stands to the S side facing the client, own feet spread apart for stability, with toes pointing into the angle between the seats and with knees ready to prop up a collapsing S knee. For a L hemiplegic client moving to a seat on their left, the helper's nearside arm tucks under the N arm and outside arm embraces over the S arm to exert pressure into the chest wall below the scapula. For a client with R hemiplegia, the procedure is vice versa.

- Keeping head and shoulders well away to the S side, the helper leans over the S shoulder (avoiding head contact) to enable the client to move their CoG forwards normally over their feet,

- Giving a slight forward pull, lift and swing-round into the second seat in order to initiate the automatic response sequence of part-rise, swivel, sit (see Fig. 6.6).

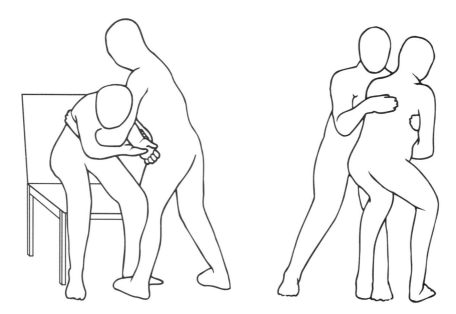

Fig. 6.6

Persevere: it may seem awkward at first but the client will quickly progress to requiring less and less assistance until independent transferring is achieved (see Fig. 6.7).

Positioning hazards

No one position should be maintained for long. Static postures are not normal, and if sustained for longer than an hour or so will result in stereotyped (abnormal) reflex patterns developing – and pressure sores.

Small natural movements are beneficial: lifting and replacing feet, wriggling, transferring weight from one buttock to the other and back again, turning and twisting to reach for things. So encourage clients to shift about a bit in the chair, how to regain the advantageous positions and to ask for assistance to do so if necessary. Stroke survivors need to be aware of the position of their S limbs too, by looking for them if sensation is faulty. Dangling hands and arms result in gravitational oedema (swelling) and possible trauma (trapped under body, grazed against furniture). Inversion (twisting inwards) of the S foot leads to chronic inflammation and probable spraining of the ankle joint.

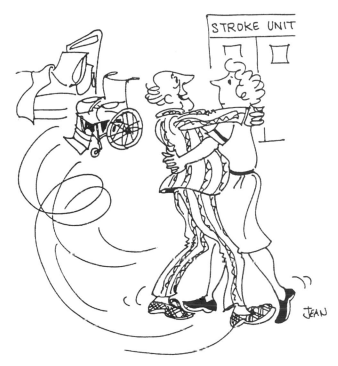

Fig. 6.7 'Did you say "Hang on and Pivot"?'

Subcortical stimulation

When a stroke survivor is apparently unable to make a planned move or to move appropriately to an instruction ('lean forwards', 'take a step'), this could be due to cognitive disruption such as a dyspraxia or to more general sensorimotor impairment. It is likely, however, that appropriate movement sequences can still be initiated by stimulating the subcortical systems directly to gain an 'automatic' response, using non-verbal sensory pathways (also valuable in working with some language-impaired clients):

Visual clues: use gesture and body-language; beckon someone to come forward, to get up; point to direct attention; hold out your hands or an object (towel, book) just out of reach (but casually!) to encourage forward leaning, and so on.

Tactile (touch) cues: a light touch on an arm to gain attention; gentle pressure behind a shoulder for turning.

Proprioceptive cueing: use the facilitation techniques, using keypoints, to gain a required action, as described in the next section.

Facilitating 'normal' movement   Facilitation is where handling proceeds into assisted dynamic movement, both simple and complex. By introducing subtle changes in the relationship between the CoG and the BoS, whole sequences of normal 'automatic' responses can usually be stimulated. It is the basis for all skilled intervention: abnormal movement patterns can be inhibited and naturally recovering movement, together with any developing re-learned movement, can be co-ordinated and manipulated into normal functional activity.

Remember that you are 'guiding' the action, not asking clients to try to do this – it is the subcortical 'automatic', instinctive, responses caught in the stroke disorganization that you are aiming to recover from them. Practice on friends/family/colleagues first to get the feel of it and 'how far to go' (only far enough to elicit the expected response).

Support firmly but gently where and when necessary for movement through and against gravity, but do not give more support than is absolutely essential at any stage. Otherwise the recipient will only learn dependence on assistance from others. The guiding is by hand or fingertip pressure at identified 'keypoints' on the body:

Keypoints   The 'automatic' alignment, righting and equilibrium responses can be stimulated by the skilful direction of body movement controlled through certain points on the human frame.

Central keypoint:
- Mid-chest, back and front (the assumed CoG)

Threatening disturbance of a person's CoG, by applying pressure at the central keypoint (front or back), will facilitate automatic postural adjustments (including limb movements for equilibrium if the threat persists) in the recipient *if* these responses are present.

For example: In sitting, sustained forward pressure from behind the central keypoint (with fingertips or a gentle hand) will initiate the rising-to-standing sequence (don't explain first – a recipient 'in the know' will merely end up with their face on their knees). In standing, this keypoint pressure will result in stepping forwards (if pre-warned, the person will merely push backwards against you).

Proximal keypoints:
- Shoulders
- Hips

Stand alongside or behind the recipient with a gentle but firm grasp at the shoulders or at each side of the pelvis (try both ways in turn and use whichever works best), and apply forward pressure to propel the person forwards. Turning can be stimulated and controlled, and gentle backward pulling will initiate stepping backwards. Weight-transference, stepping sideways, and correction of undue inward/outward rotation at the hip during walking can also be manipulated.

Use weight transference to facilitate normal locomotion when the client has achieved self-controlled standing and stepping balance (described below).

Peripheral keypoints:
- Limb joints

Used mainly to direct ongoing movement or to intercept unwanted activity, which must be prevented by using the other hand to anticipate and intercept it appropriately.

For example: pressure from a hand behind the S elbow will prevent the S arm collapsing into flexion (bending) if bodyweight needs to be taken through a straight arm for supported standing, pushing, walking. Fingertip patting or hand pressure over the patella (kneecap) can stimulate the bracing, or prevent the collapsing, of a S knee.

Contact dancing (best ballroom style – particularly jive) is a good example of facilitation. Every turn and twist is directed, intercepted, redirected and controlled from the keypoints at fingers, shoulders, hips, by an expert partner.

As recovery and re-learning progresses, less and less physical help will be needed until certain, if not all, basic moves are in place again, depending on the severity of the stroke.

Re-educating balance

Most people experience difficulty with balance after a stroke, because their automatic postural adjustments in relation to gravity are impaired or impoverished by altered muscle tone and possible denervation of muscle tissue on the S side. In a few really severe cases this remains a problem; however, others should regain a satisfactory level of control after a few days' work at each stage (sitting, standing, stepping and walking), given the right assistance at the right time. Without this input, even lengthy and intensive rehabilitation will not fully eradicate the compensatory 'snatch/grab and hang-on' habits acquired for self-preservation.

Sitting balance

As for all movement, this is best achieved by consistent control and facilitation during familiar daily functional activity. Begin at the beginning! Getting up every morning to sit on the side of the bed; getting washed and dressed while sitting on the side of the bed; transferring into a chair or wheelchair for the rest of the day's activity; reversing the sequences to end the day by getting back into bed again.

Sitting on the side of the bed

Once the client is sitting with feet on the floor, the helper sits alongside the S side with nearside arm ready round the back to catch any sudden lurch (don't make contact – otherwise client will lean into you). Helper's offside arm is free to protect any forward fall. Allow for (and encourage) a little natural sway in all directions: this in itself may be enough to re-awaken normal postural control mechanisms.

Reminders will be needed frequently at first ('right/left a bit', 'a bit more', 'lean more to me' etc.). Actively intervene with a nudge in the appropriate direction only when the client's CoG is reaching an irretrievable point beyond their BoS (going, still going, Oops! catch, guide back into a state of balance again) and repeat.

The client needs to really concentrate on gaining balance control in sitting, so avoid and discourage chatting or distracting until this is achieved.

If the client persistently topples to both sides, then a second helper is needed to sit alongside the N side. Some stroke survivors seem determined to push themselves over by shoving with their N arm and leg, discussed at the end of this section.

Washing and dressing are part of the balance re-learning programme; when they involve sitting on the side of the bed, even when assisted or actually carried out by the helper/s while the recipient concentrates on maintaining equilibrium. Just picking someone up and propping them in an armchair to hold them up will never restore their ability to cope with even the most basic activities. Neuro-physiotherapists are often thought to be idling their time away on the wards (so I've been told!), sitting down on the job instead of behaving like gym instructors in the privacy of their own departments. They are of course working extremely hard to re-develop a client's postural control against gravity in an effective environment – the first and most vital stage of rehabilitation which demands profound concentration by all parties.

Once the client's sitting balance can be sustained while other things are going on, the individual can begin to participate actively (with self-control over their equilibrium still taking priority) until the goal is reached – automatic postural control, regardless of distracting influences (the first step towards optimum independence).

Sitting to standing and vice versa

This should be facilitated as part of the washing/dressing procedure in order to cleanse personal nether regions, to pull up underpants, tights, trousers, and for toileting. Hip-hitching to the edge of the seat and the body-clasp used for swivel transfers (without the 'swivel') will make this very easy for everyone. The helper needs to keep own body and head well clear to the S side while bringing the client's CoG forwards over their feet, then a little hoist forwards and upwards (supporting the S knee with own knee) will result in standing.

Lame dogma:
- 'Clasp your hands together and push down towards the floor' – sometimes including 'keep your head down':

This is often the advice given to people struggling to stand up. Try doing this yourself – it doesn't work and could also put unnecessary 'pulling' stress on a vulnerable S shoulder.

Sitting down from standing is not a positive action, it is merely a controlled relaxation from the standing position. Keep the client's CoG forwards over their knees (supported by helper's knees) throughout, guiding from keypoints as appropriate, as the rump eases backwards over the seat. Encourage the individual to glance behind (to the S side first) to assess for themselves the correct moment for the final relaxation down into sitting. If explicit instruction is needed, you could prompt with 'lean forward and feel for the back of the chair with your backside!'

Performed properly, standing up/sitting down is an excellent exercise for ongoing dynamic activity. Performed frequently, it is also a strengthening exercise for the thighs, buttocks and back muscles (try it, slowly, up to five times, with hands resting on your thighs to feel them working).

Standing balance

As rising and re-sitting improves, more time can be spent establishing dynamic postural control in standing – just a few seconds between moves (perhaps before sitting down) will contribute to progress.

With feet a little apart (to give a broader BoS) and the helper standing to the stroke side (as always) or sitting in front (easier to control the action at the hips), introduce turning from the waist to look around to either side and behind. Allow natural sway: do not touch unless intervention (with a nudge or a little pull on clothing) is required to prevent overshooting. Progress to reaching forwards, sideways, down, for articles (always make movement purposeful and task specific); this will involve natural 'transference of weight' from leg to leg and also between toes and heels.

Independent standing, stepping and/or walking is readily achievable by the vast majority of stroke-disabled people. Many who appear to be severely affected are denied the opportunity to achieve these goals because these early routines are not adhered to or are not implemented for long enough. Always look to the next stage at each stage: giving up will condemn a stroke survivor to a chairbound existence, usually quite unnecessarily (iatrogenically disabled). Most people will regain partial or even fully independent mobility (with a walking aid if necessary) quite quickly, given this background of consistent and knowledgeable assistance.

Stepping and walking

Once automatic balance reactions in weight-transference are established, 'stepping' is introduced by the physiotherapist who will facilitate normal gait patterns for progression into 'walking'.

Lame dogmas:
- Walking is top priority
- Anyone can teach walking

No walking isn't top priority – regaining self-controlled balance in all situations is Top Priority. No one should be hauled to their feet to stumble around between two helpers (or one and a Zimmer frame). This does not re-educate 'walking', it only teaches dependence on others and a compensatory abnormal, disabled gait. It also fills people with fear (thereby increasing reflex activity and spasticity) because they are not in control of their own equilibrium. It disables people.

Starting to walk, the use of walking aids, managing steps and stairs are activities that should be initiated and directed by the physiotherapist. Some relevant protocols are described briefly in the section on professional strategies – the procedures should be used (with care and understanding) only if physiotherapy services are not available for the client.

In all these procedures, less and less physical assistance will be required as postural control improves, confidence and competent progress towards more independent activity are achieved.

Lame dogma:
- 'We haven't got time for all this.'

It takes very little extra time to guide and protect normal movement patterns in all the daily routines, whether on a ward or elsewhere. The time spent is rapidly made up as clients will fast become more self-sufficient, thereby requiring much less time than would be spent on doing everything for them.

'Pushers'

These are people – often with a L hemiplegia, sensory 'loss' and sometimes with perceptual 'unilateral neglect' – who forcefully and persistently push themselves off-balance to their S side. Their righting reactions and protective reflexes are non-functioning on the S side, so any disturbance that stimulates these automatic reactions produces a one-sided – the N side – response. Aware that they are toppling over, these clients frantically brace themselves to prevent it, but only the musculature on the N side responds; this of course pushes them further over, so they try even harder to brace themselves to prevent it happening.

If someone else tries to push these clients upright again, this causes greater effort in bracing against the extra (felt as threatening) push. The N hand desperately tries to remedy the situation by clutching and pulling at anything within reach, but this only adds to a no-win situation. Pulling at people or things does not give stability – think of strap-hanging in a subway train – but leaning on something can help.

Help with sitting

A second helper is required, sitting alongside the N side and insisting on close shoulder and hip contact until upright posture can be sustained. Then move away gently and encourage the client to self-support on the bed, using the N arm/hand to lean on but not to push with. This is an important factor for people with the 'pusher' syndrome but not for any other stroke sufferers; pushers have to learn to self-support to their N side as well. The primary helper should lean away from the S side, discouraging body contact, while pursuing the task on hand (washing, dressing etc.). If pushing-over to the S side re-occurs, the second helper can prompt with 'lean into me again' or 'take/lean your weight on your N hand'. A full-length mirror in front also helps with feedback for self-righting skills.

Help with standing

Two helpers are needed, as above, one standing shoulder-to-shoulder and hip-to-hip on the N side and insisting on contact at both points ('lean towards me don't go away, shoulder to shoulder, remember?') but not allowing any hand or arm support at all (a helping hand will be pulled and pumped up and down). Alternatively, stand the client alongside a bed or table to the N side with the flat of N hand on the bed or table to allow support without pulling.

The primary helper on the S side gives straight-arm support to the S arm using the hand-to-hand hold, making sure the elbow is as straight as possible, to directly stimulate a supporting reaction from the S side of the body. Prompt 'Push! My hand is a walking stick, lean on it' (see Fig. 6.8). It may even be advantageous to give a walking stick for use in the N hand provided the client has learn to lean on to it, and the physiotherapist agrees.

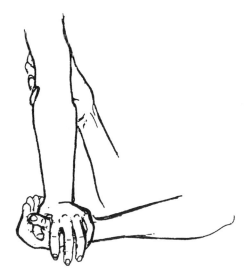

Fig. 6.8 Helper's hand-to-hand hold for S arm.

Persevere, this problem can be overcome! If it is not dealt with early, the poor client will never be able to stand, transfer between seats, let alone walk, without maximum assistance regardless of any recovering mobility. Pushers are frequently found in the clutches of a struggling carer, an illicit walking stick in N hand waving in the air as they both fight to regain equilibrium.

Wheelchair management

Some people will have to settle for mobility on wheels, either because their balance is irretrievably impaired or because they are assessed to be at risk for living alone or unattended for long periods, or their walking ability is limited to short distances.

Ambulation can be delayed by supplying a wheelchair too quickly – it is the easy option for impatient people. However, if local policy favours early provision, then the chair must be matched to the client and effective rules imposed.

Even for short trips (to the toilet, the dayroom, the dining table) the S foot must be firmly on the footplate, heel well down, not scooped up by the N leg (which reinforces the abnormal reflex patterns of S knee extension with outward rotation at the hip and ankle inversion and also reinforces 'non-use' of the S limb into the sensorimotor system).

Scudding around self-propelled by the N hand and foot requires weightbearing on the N side (try it) which unleashes the reflex patterns on the S side. Customized seat-height and constant monitoring of posture and position may help but does not adequately prevent the reflexes from happening.

Tyres must be kept pumped up and the brakes checked regularly. If tyres are flabby, the brakes won't be effective anyway.

At kerbs and steps the chair goes forwards up and backwards down, otherwise the occupant is tipped out.

Lame dogma:
- An extended brake lever on the S side (for use by the N hand) encourages transference of weight to the S side and is 'A Good Thing'.

Wrong! An extended brake lever obstructs transferring to another seat/toilet/bed to the S side, and gets knocked by the footplate every time it is swung back, thereby releasing the brake at a critical moment. Using an extended lever with the N hand forces the trunk into the traditional twisty reflex posture and tips even more weight on to the N leg. Try it: as the R arm crosses over to reach a lever on the left, the L shoulder swings backwards and the L hip hitches up to shorten the trunk on that side – and vice versa. A single brake lever fitted to the N side which controls both brakes is preferable by far.

Professional strategies

Stroke management should be pragmatic and correlate new knowledge with new concepts and theoretical approaches as these are formulated and expanded. Clinicians need to be able to develop – and discard when irrelevant – strategies and practices by heuristic application and evaluation.

That we are manipulating mature brain activity with every intervention is probably the most significant discovery. The corollary is especially important – that everyone working with a stroke survivor has the same influence and that all the movement involved in a survivor's everyday activities is affected. The evidence relating to cognition and movement has been around for some time, but the majority of health professionals seem unaware of the implications. Physiotherapists, as members of the only 'hands-on' profession whose core expertise is designed to promote the restoration of physical movement and mobility, have to be particularly aware of the facts. We are all involved in trophic engineering whatever we do. We can further disable our clients by uninformed intervention and by failing to communicate to others working with neurologically impaired people the issues regarding neuromuscular plasticity, physiological and cognitive stressing.

Techniques used in stroke rehabilitation need to be learned from experienced practitioners in workshop situations, with application and effect clearly understood. No two stroke survivors will have the same set of problems, nor will they respond in the same way to the same techniques. Many, indeed, will not benefit from any of the currently recognized approaches. Bear in mind too that the use of inflatable splints, the motor relearning programme (Carr & Shepherd, 1987), 'Bobath' (now teaching techniques developed by Lynch), gymnastic balls, and all the others – these approaches are not mutually exclusive. Try everything that seems applicable at the time, mix and match them, try something else. If it doesn't work, don't use it!

This principle applies to all techniques and strategies. Return to them later if they still seem appropriate. Versatility is vital – have a wide repertoire and sufficient knowledge to invent your own when all else fails.

Familiar task-specific activities provide the platform for any intervention. Unrelated 'exercises' and those aimed at component parts of a movement pattern in isolation (ankle-dorsiflexion today) can no longer be justified, except maybe in the later stages of recovery when a particular skill or activity needs polishing.

This section describes some fundamental strategies as a baseline for more sophisticated approaches. As previously, the term 'helper' is used indiscriminately (a physiotherapist is not always available), but any new activity should be designed and supervised by a physiotherapist. All progress made in performance (independent transfers, for instance) needs to be adopted into the familiar activities of daily living for cognitive 'carry-over', as schema for motor behaviour in all situations are rebuilt.

Subcortical stimulation, discussed earlier, also enables accurate appraisal of ongoing performance, as recovery can be related to the sustained use or re-acquisition of more normal patterns of 'automatic' motor behaviour – the degree of re-learning of sensorimotor adaptability – in both structured and unstructured situations.

Indirect exercise

This relies on positioning the individual so that bodyweight is distributed through the proximal joints on the S side, and then on demanding activity from the N limbs (the only time that non-functional exercise is recommended!). This will elicit automatic movement responses on the S side, involving equilibrium reactions and transference of weight, and will also stimulate selective adjustments in position. A second helper may be needed to facilitate and control these to prevent unwanted reflex activity. It is also a subtle way to bombard hypotonic or catabolized muscle tissue in order to stress and rebuild activity for better quality of movement and improved performance.

For example, with the client:

- Lying on the S side (on flat of scapula, not point of shoulder), exercises with the N arm and leg will generate postural equilibrium adjustments in the S side trunk and limbs;
- Sitting with feet on the floor, lifting and placing games with the N foot;
- Perch-sitting on the edge of a raised bed, plinth or table, turned slightly to the N side with N hip hitched further back and N leg swinging free (foot well clear of the floor), this position will leave the S leg (S foot firmly on the floor) in position to support bodyweight during games and exercises with N arm, or both if possible, which involve reaching and placing. This stimulates dynamic bracing and adjusting activity in the S leg, buttock and trunk.

'Pushers'

This problem seems to affect mostly those with a L hemiplegia, often with apparently good movement in the S leg, and is often associated with sensory impairment in the S limbs and/or perceptual unilateral neglect. It may be caused by a 'glitch' in the sensorimotor processing which fails to recruit the protective supporting reactions on the S side, whilst failing to control appropriate equilibrium activity on the N side (the N upper limb tends to fly up instead of supporting down). It can be overcome by stimulating supporting reactions from the S side only, whilst encouraging appropriate leaning and supporting activity on the N side. Work through progressively with the client:

(1)   Sitting on a raised plinth/table with both feet clear of the ground to prevent pushing with the N leg, for balance activities. Give a supporting surface (pillows, small stool) on the plinth for S hand or forearm only.

(2)   Perch-sitting activities with S foot on the floor, as for 'indirect exercise'.
(3)   Standing with second helper on N side to give positive sensory alignment for hip/shoulder but no other hands-on input while the S hand/arm/shoulder is facilitated to support bodyweight; use either the hand-to-hand hold or a stable surface at an appropriate height (preferable).
(4)   Walking using the same strategy. Progress to walking between two stable surfaces (NOT parallel bars, these only reinforce the pulling-up instead of the leaning-down-on action) with the N hand resting on the other, supporting if required, but moving forwarding appropriately with alternate steps.

Giving a stick for use in the N hand before effective gait is established (as above) will only reinforce the original problem. These are the people who wave their sticks in the air while falling over (they are trying to pull on them instead of lean on them). But a rollator can be helpful in the meantime if the S upper limb is functional and its supporting activity is carefully monitored (to avoid any grasp/flex activity).

Variable-height plinths, tables and beds

Surface heights introduce a great range of dynamic activity for early or severely handicapped clients, and for progress to independent balance and gait. Surface heights can be adjusted to the requisite needs of each individual, to maximize normal movement responses for ongoing functional activity.

Supporting reactions can be stimulated in S limbs by giving a facility for forearm or straight arm support on one plinth while sitting or kneeling on the other, and in standing. This also brings in the secondary systems of presynaptic inhibition to abort or overcome primitive reflex patterns.

Rising to stand and sitting again can be relearned by altering the relative heights of plinths to accommodate forearm or straight-arm support on the second surface. This encourages appropriate shifting of the CoG in relation to the BoS. And 'transfers' can be taught with less effort needed by all concerned (see Fig. 6.9).

Standing balance can be facilitated between two plinths at hip-height and far enough apart (up to 6 in clearance) to allow natural sway; overshooting is halted by contact with a plinth to give feedback. This frees the therapist to inhibit abnormal patterns by facilitating postural dynamics from top to toe.

Transference of weight as a prelude to stepping and walking is facilitated the same way; as the CoG shifts over the S leg, you should encourage the client to gently ease the N foot off the ground, and repeat the sequence vice versa. (Always start with bodyweight over the S side, N leg active first, to inhibit reflex action and stimulate a normal response.)

Lame dogma:
● 'Parallel bars help people to walk again.'

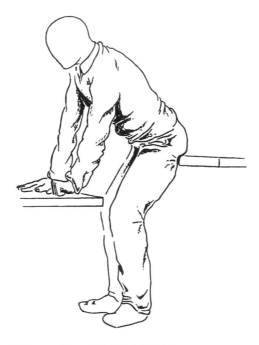

Fig. 6.9 Rising to stand between two variable height plinths.

Nonsense! Parallel bars teach people to grab and pull instead of supporting themselves, they nullify any natural automatic postural adjustments vital to self-controlled balance and therefore deny progress to any independent activity. They also trigger and then reinforce the grasp and flexion reflexes in the S upper limb, and encourage compensatory weightbearing to the N side which further releases abnormal reflex activity. Parallel bars disable – rather than enable – stroke survivors.

Stepping: once the natural transferring of bodyweight from foot to foot is achieved, it is simple to progress to stepping forwards and backwards between the two plinths, using supporting reactions in the S arm (the plinth on the S side can be raised to allow forearm support if the hand is vulnerable) to further inhibit reflex activity and to gain natural alternate arm/leg swing. Most clients require this interim stage to gain confidence in their own ability to cope with the dynamic postural control against the gravity involved in locomotion, with BoS reduced (to single foot and less as it alternates between toe and heel for swing-through, phasing, etc.) in conjunction with the ongoing disturbances of their CoG.

If stability and dynamic postural control is already well established, a brief stepping procedure serves as a simple warm-up to actual locomotion until walking itself has regained sensorimotor adaptability.

Progress to stepping alongside a single plinth on the S side. Those who needed to walk with a stick before the stroke will, of course, need to use one afterwards, in the N hand for optimum security. Stroke-disabled clients always need to step 'best foot first' to abort reflex activity in the S side and to reawaken reciprocal innervation. It is a fundamental rule but extraordinarily difficult for some clients to do 'normally'. It requires physiological stressing and controlled dynamic true transference of weight over the S leg which may be subject to latent extensor reflex activity and will flex at the hip.

- Begin by facilitating the client's CoG diagonally forwards and sideways, over and on to the S leg, before guiding just one step forwards with the N leg.
- Then control the CoG as it moves over for weightbearing on the N leg, while monitoring the reciprocal relaxation of the S leg (allowing a sharp swing back over the N leg will undo the benefits gained).
- Ensure equilibrium is regained before the process is repeated to allow the N leg to step back into place, again with bodyweight finally distributed equally between both feet.
- Repeat with stepping backwards with the N leg only, too, at this stage, until fluent stepping with the N leg and the appropriate postural adjustments are satisfactorily achieved.
- Once gained, facilitate a natural follow-through with the S leg and another controlled step with the N leg and then repeat stepping backwards.
- Equilibrium must be controlled throughout – if the performance snarls up, go back a stage and allow the client to rest (in a comfortable reflex-inhibiting position, sitting or lying) before continuing.
- Progress to stepping in a cleared space, with a helper to offer support to the S side if it is required.

Walking strategies

Gait pattern can be facilitated from proximal keypoints. Ensure that any trunk distortion is corrected and stop for a rest period (facilitating easy sitting/lying on couch as needed in a comfortable reflex-inhibiting position) if tone is rising in S side musculature.

If independent walking is faulty to start with, then supply an appropriate walking-aid before compensatory abnormal patterns kick in. 'Normal' gait using an aid will physiologically stress normal gait patterns; abnormal gait without any aid will obviously reinforce abnormal patterns.

A rollator gives useful non-reflexive functional activity to a recovering S hand and arm; weight-bearing through the upper limb utilizes the secondary systems of presynaptic inhibition and will improve performance generally. It is also beneficial for ataxic gait. Fitted with forearm supports, a rollator can be used by clients with poor upper limb function. Never supply a Zimmer-type frame unless the client has full use of the S arm and hand and can walk well without but requires the support for other reasons (arthritis, frail elderly, etc.). A Zimmer reinforces the grasp reflex in a S hand and can trigger a full flexor-withdrawal pattern in the arm with hyper-reflexive extension in the trunk as the frame is picked up for each step forwards.

Include turning and manoeuvring around obstacles, opening and closing doors, slopes, and uneven surfaces, as soon as possible.

Steps and stairs strategies

These need to be added early into the walking programme to exploit any 'automatic' resources still uncontaminated by acquired handicaps such as fear of falling or a general loss of confidence (a kerb-height dais, large enough to take a rollator, is a very useful piece of equipment).

A helper should stand below the client, hand ready to firm a collapsible knee and to facilitate hip/knee flexion. If hypotonic or partially-denervated musculature remains a problem, start with N leg up, S leg down, to improve control of the supporting reaction in the S leg – but prevent hyper-extension at the S knee. With a single stair rail only, sideways stepping up and down may be helpful.

General activities

Physiotherapy should also progress movement re-education into a wide variety of functional situations in different locations, to ensure carry-over of relearned skills. For instance, facilitated walking into the next department for a follow-on occupational therapy session (instead of in the structured environment of the gym before being bundled into a wheelchair for portered transit) will help to build action schemata. Taking a client to the toilet and facilitating their movement skills with undoing clothing, reaching, sitting and rising, is rehabilitation and must be seen as such.

Home visits/community

If possible, you should accompany a client on an early trip home in order to gain insight into the levels of performance and coping skills that will be required – and continue to facilitate 'normal' movement during the visit, wherever appropriate, once the social niceties have been attended to.

Physiotherapy input on these occasions can also establish the need to allow for ongoing progress where this is predicted; a downstairs toilet or a stairlift may be unnecessary if the client is on the way to achieving successful stairclimbing.

Assessments and outcomes

No infallible systems have been devised so far, although there are many promising developments being considered. The medical profession favours two clinical indicators to poor recovery:

(1)   Coma lasting longer then one week. But this often only indicates a more oedematous reaction to the acute event; a remarkably good recovery can

follow as the oedema subsides, particularly if general nursing care follows a proper stroke management policy in handling and positioning.
(2) Incontinence lasting longer than one week. This could indicate a lesion involving more complex CNS control systems, but is more likely to be the result of poor continence management. Call in the continence advisor, early. In any case, rehabilitation should continue, as the potential for recovery in all the other systems may well be unaffected. Increasing dynamic activity itself will stimulate the relevant musculature, both striated and smooth, and may even re-activate the continence control systems.

For example, an elderly woman with an apparently dense R 'hemiparesis' was nursed on an elderly care ward for three weeks until the consultant decreed her discharge into long-term care in a nursing home, 'As she will never be continent/ walk/talk again and will probably die in a couple of months'. Her family insisted on her transfer to a nearby stroke unit, where she made an excellent recovery within two months and is now driving again, doing the *Telegraph* crossword and conversing fluently with just an occasional word-finding problem.

There are two biomechanical indicators for good recovery:

(1) Up and walking within three weeks (!)
(2) Walking a measured distance in a given time ('normal' average speed).

Mulder *et al.* (1994) suggest that biomechanical parameters are less relevant to the prediction of ability in daily-life activities than those based on the cognitive control of motor behaviour. Mulder submits that assessment of performance should relate to the three stages of recovery (here repeated from the previous chapter):

(1) the cognitive stage in which the learner makes an initial approximation to the skill, based on tacit knowledge, observation and instruction;
(2) the associative stage in which performance is refined through the elimination of errors;
(3) the autonomous stage in which skilled performance is well-established.

Shifts in these motor control processes across time could give an objective indication of recovery: good recovery being defined as the recovery of sensorimotor adaptability (the re-automatisation of motor tasks). This seems to be a far more realistic route for developing assessment procedures than the application of a battery of tests for non-task-oriented abilities (or in artificial tasks) or for the components of a movement unrelated to actual activity.

Summary

Neurophysiotherapy enables people to achieve their maximum potential for the recovery of movement skills in functional performance – or the achievement of acceptable alternative strategies for coping – in partnership with the client, family, carers and all members of the healthcare team. Listed below are some points to remember:

- Good recovery should never be confused with 'back-to-normal'. It should be assessed in terms of optimal restoration to functional health status, including leisure and pleasure activity.
- Techniques should be used with imagination and pragmatism, and be customized to the individual. For example, mat exercises for the elderly and arthritic are inappropriate – use a large low plinth even for practising 'up from falling' until they have mastered the principle.
- Interventions should never cause pain (I once overheard a client say 'I know it's doing me good because it hurts', as he hauled his S arm up into full elevation). Pain means trauma.
- Mobility does not depend on walking – it is to do with getting around as efficiently as possible.
- Dependence on other people for some or all of the activities of daily living does not signify failure either for the individual or the team, provided that the rehabilitation has been sufficiently knowledgeable and extensive, and that preparation for possible outcomes has been introduced effectively into the programme.
- Independence is a goal but not the only goal for the stroke survivor. Quality of life after a stroke has to be the main objective for all concerned.
- Iatrogenesis should never be an issue.

References

Carr, J.H. & Shepherd, R.B. (1987) *A Motor Relearning Programme for Stroke.* Heinemann Medical, Oxford.

Laidler, P. (1994) *Stroke Rehabilitation: Structure and Strategy.* Stanley Thornes, Cheltenham.

Mulder, T. (1992) Current ideas on motor control and learning: implications for therapy. In *Spinal Cord Dysfunction, Intervention and Treatment*, Vol. 11 (L.S. Illis, ed.), pp. 187–209. Oxford University Press, Oxford.

Mulder, T., Pauwels, J. & Nienhuis, B. (1994) Motor recovery following stroke: towards a disability-oriented assessment of motor dysfunctions. In *Physiotherapy in Stroke Management: Proceedings of WCPT/Europe Conference* (M. Harrison, ed.), pp. 275–82. Churchill Livingstone, Edinburgh.

Relevant reading

Ada, L. & Canning, C. (1990) *Key Issues in Neurological Physiotherapy.* Heinemann, London.

Davies, P.M. (1985) *Steps to Follow: A Guide to the Treatment of Adult Hemiplegia.* Springer-Verlag, Berlin.

Chapter 7
Speech and Language Problems Following Stroke

Jane Marshall

Dysphasia

Dysphasia, or aphasia, is a language disorder arising from neurological impairment, usually as a result of damage in the left side of the brain. However, there are rare cases arising from right sided lesions (sometimes termed 'crossed aphasia'). Approximately 30% of stroke patients acquire a lasting dysphasia (Bonita & Anderson, 1983). Technically, aphasia means total loss of language and dysphasia partial loss. However, the terms tend to be used interchangeably.

Dysphasia impairs all aspects of language, e.g. speech production, comprehension, reading and writing; it may also affect the person's gestures and the use of drawing to communicate. Dysphasia is different from general cognitive impairment and does not interfere with the person's ability to plan their lives, have opinions, remember, think and imagine   as can be demonstrated by non-verbal tests of memory and reasoning.

One of the most puzzling features of dysphasia is its extreme variability, both in terms of the severity and nature of the disorder, as illustrated in Table 7.1.

Speaker 1 has a particular difficulty thinking of the words he wants to use, although is speech is grammatical. He has *anomia*, a word finding problem, and has a number of strategies to help overcome this problem: he can draw his ideas or use gestures and carry on a conversation. Although he often cannot produce words independently, he can repeat them; so when the therapist says 'navy', he repeats this word in response.

Speaker 2 accesses key nouns more successfully than the first speaker. However, her speech almost completely lacks grammar or is *agrammatic*: there are no sentences, few grammatical words (like 'is' and 'of') and no verbs. She is good at listing objects, but very poor at conveying what she has been doing; she seems quite good at understanding sentences even though she cannot produce appropriate responses to the therapist's questions. However, sentence comprehension is not always preserved in agrammatism.

Speaker 3 has *jargon aphasia*: speech is fluent, even copious, but the meaning is

Table. 7.1 Examples of dysphasic speech.

Speaker 1 (RS)

RS: 'Where we are it's a . . . not a house . . . you know when there's only one . . . er, no up . . . oh, I know what it is . . . it drives me mad' (draws a picture of a bungalow).

RS: 'I used to be in the . . . here' (writes 1939 – 1945).

Therapist: offers 'navy'?

RS: 'No, not the navy . . . but (gestures marching) you know, one two, one two.'

(unpublished clinical data)

Speaker 2 (EM)

Therapist: 'How was your Christmas?'

EM: 'Fine, fine . . . um, New Year and Christmas, um . . . Peter.'

Therapist: 'Did he come to you?'

EM: 'No (gestures away from self) . . . yes.'

Therapist: 'What did you eat?'

EM: 'Turkey and stuffing, potatoes, cauliflower, sprouts, carrots, swede.'

Therapist: 'And what presents did you give?'

EM: 'um Margaret . . . um jumper and trousers and um Steven . . . its um CD

(from Marshall, J. 1994, unpublished Ph.D thesis)

Speaker 3 (RG)

(Describing a picture of a doctor examining a woman with a broken leg with probable target words given in parenthesis)

Woman sitting on the /ops/ (wheelchair) is er sitting in front of a doctor . . . um he's got his /sekops/ (stethoscope) on . . . er and he got a list of fictions (medical notes) of what's wrong with her she got a . . . super walk (crutch) to support her when she gets out of the /ko ke/ (wheelchair) her legs are on a . . . /snriand/ (footplate) and the whole of the right /les/ (leg) is covered in cement (plaster)

(from Marshall *et al.* 1996)

very difficult to determine, mainly because of the proliferation of errors and the use of nonwords or *neologisms*. The sample shows that Speaker 3's neologisms are not consistent, i.e. his first attempt at wheel chair is /ops/ ('orps') and his second is /ko ke/ ('korker'). Like the other dysphasic speakers, RG has some strengths: on the whole his speech is grammatical and, unlike EM, he is quite skilled in accessing verbs; and some phrases also express elements of the target word (such as 'super walk' for 'crutch').

To understand the different manifestations of aphasia, remember that some variations seem to relate to the site of the lesion. For example, damage to the left frontal areas of the brain tends to produce Speaker 2's nonfluent speech, while more posterior damage is associated with the fluent but disordered output of Speaker 3 (Damasio, 1991). However, there are exceptions to these patterns, and subjects with apparently similar lesions may display quite different language skills.

Poor understanding of language–brain relationships has resulted in alternative approaches to the study of dysphasia: e.g. the information processing approach (Ellis & Young, 1996, Kay *et al.*, 1992), where clinicians employ schematic models of how the brain produces or comprehends language to interpret dysphasic symptoms. This approach attempts to explain the subjects' problems in terms of specific points of failure within an abstract language system, as illustrated in the following sections.

Problems producing single words

Word finding problems are a common, if not ubiquitous, symptom of most types of dysphasia, as shown by Speaker 1 (Table 7.1). The simple model below based on work by Ellis and Young (1996) explained more about anomia by considering how the language system normally accesses words.

This model suggests that word production entails three broad stages: the first accesses the *semantic* representation of the target as a cluster of features which make up the meaning of the word. For example, for 'cup' the features would include: item of crockery, open container, with handle, for drinking. The second

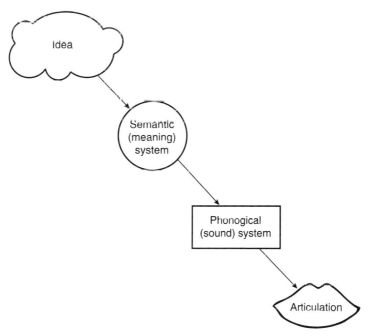

Fig. 7.1 A model of word production.

stage accesses the *phonology*, or sound, of the word; and the final stage articulates the word.

In anomia, this word production system has broken down at a number of stages. Some anomic people have a deficit at the semantic level (Howard and Orchard-Lisle, 1984; Hillis *et al.*, 1990; Beaton *et al.*, 1997). These people can no longer access full information about the meaning of words. One sign of this may be semantic errors, where the person produces a word that is close in meaning to the intended target – so instead of 'cup' they may say 'plate'. In Table 7.1, Speaker 3 made an error of this type, where 'plaster' was called 'cement'. Furthermore, RG, like other people who make semantic errors, is usually unaware of his mistakes.

People with semantic problems may also find it difficult to use strategies such as writing to overcome their problem, as this also requires semantic processing. The person may even be unable to draw or gesture the target, because of a lack of semantic information needed to stimulate these alternative forms of output. Above all, a semantic deficit is signalled by parallel difficulties in understanding words, since just one meaning system serves production and comprehension.

Other individuals have problems accessing the phonologies of words, even though their semantic information is intact (Kay & Ellis, 1987). People with this level of impairment know the meaning of the words that they want to speak and may even be able to impart some of this information, via circumlocution. Thus, Speaker 1 (Table 7.1) was unable to access 'bungalow' but could say that it had 'only one' and 'no up'. Similarly, the person studied by Kay & Ellis (1987) could not say 'snowman' but could say: 'it's cold ... it's a man ... cold ... frozen'. If the problem is purely in accessing phonology, alternative modes of output may be relatively intact. For example, the person may be able to write words with some success and may have some understanding of speech.

People with semantic or phonological deficits are often able to produce a blocked word if they are provided with a cue. A semantic cue provides information about the meaning of a word (i.e. 'it is used in the garden', for, 'spade'). Alternatively, a phonological cue provides the first sound of the word; and a completion cue offers a lead in to the problem word (i.e. 'knife and...'). These cues can be informative about the nature of the person's deficit and suggest that words have not vanished from the person's store but are difficult to access.

Finally, word production can fail because of a deficit in the articulation stage, where the person knows both the meaning and sound of his target but cannot say the word, although he might be able to write it.

Factors affecting word production in aphasia

In aphasia, word finding problems do not affect all groups of words equally. Proper nouns (i.e. the names of people or places) are particularly problematic; and very occasionally, this problem occurs in the absence of any other aphasic deficits (Lucchelli & De Renzi, 1992). It has been argued that proper nouns are difficult because of their arbitrary nature, i.e. a person's name is simply a label, and tells us nothing about his or her personal qualities. Nevertheless, difficulties with proper names can be particularly distressing because loved ones' names can no longer be recalled, and the affected person may even be unable to supply their own name when questioned.

Other dissociations in aphasic naming have been observed. For example, uncommon words are typically more severely affected than common words. Thus Speaker 1, in Table 7.1, could say 'house' but not 'bungalow'. Another important factor may be the length of the word, in that long words may be particularly difficult (Howard *et al.*, 1984; *see* Best, 1995 for a *reverse* length effect). The meaning of the word may be important. Thus, abstract words (such as 'idea' or 'democracy') may cause particular problems (Franklin *et al.*, 1995). Finally, the person may be affected by word class, as in the example of EM in Table 7.1 who could access nouns a lot more successfully than verbs (Berndt *et al.*, 1997a).

These dissociations do not arise in all cases of aphasia, and the factors which are important often relate to the nature of the person's impairment. Thus, an individual with an articulation problem is likely to be affected by word length, while someone with a semantic deficit may well show an effect of abstractness, as mentioned above. Therefore, investigations of these factors can help to determine where the problem lies, to plan therapy and to advise friends and relatives.

Comprehension of single words

Many people with dysphasia have difficulty in understanding the words that are said to them, which could be due to a number of different reasons. Here is a simple model of how word comprehension is normally achieved:

The first process analyses the sounds in the word, e.g. that 'cup' is composed of the sounds /k/, /ʌ/ and /p/. At the next stage the word is recognized as part of the listener's vocabulary. This stage would reject a nonword, like 'brap' or an unknown foreign word. Finally, the word is fed to the semantic system, and the meaning is accessed.

According to this model there are several stages where dysphasic comprehension can break down (Franklin, 1989). Some people have problems in the preliminary stage of sound analysis. This means that they cannot tell the difference between words that sound similar, such as 'cup' and 'cut'. Others have problems with word recognition, e.g. they are unable to distinguish real words from nonwords. If these early problems are very severe, the person may seem to be deaf even though they respond appropriately to environmental sounds, such as the door bell or their dog barking. Therefore, this very specific problem with speech sounds has been termed *word deafness*. People who have word deafness usually have better reading comprehension, and a simple way to help them is to write things down.

Many people with comprehension problems have difficulties processing word meanings, either because they cannot access the semantic system, or because the

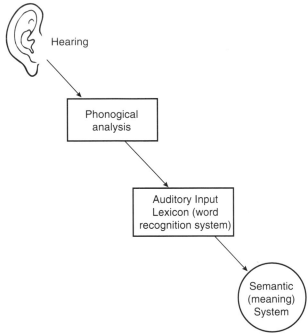

Fig. 7.2 A model of word comprehension.

system itself is damaged. The problem may be quite subtle. For example, we can test comprehension by asking the individual to point to named objects: 'show me the cup'. A person with a semantic problem may cope well with this task, providing the objects he has to choose from are quite disparate. If, however, they include a cup, a plate and a bowl, errors may occur. It seems that this person only has a very general idea of the meaning of 'cup', e.g. simply that it is an item of crockery. This information is sufficient to differentiate 'cup' from 'pencil', but not from 'bowl'. In daily life, a semantic problem might manifest in constant misunderstandings. For example, when asked to fetch the butter from the kitchen, the person may return with the jam.

As in word production, semantic disorders can generate particular problems with the understanding of abstract words (Franklin, 1989; Franklin *et al.*, 1994). This evidence accords with the intuitions that abstract words are somehow more difficult than concrete ones. However, occasionally, aphasic people are slightly *better* at processing abstract words. For example, the person studied by Marshall *et al.* (1996) was given an odd-one-out task involving either concrete or abstract words (i.e. *mud*, rock, stone; cost, value, *weight*). He was marginally better at detecting the odd-one-out in the abstract triads than in the concrete ones. Interestingly, this person also made quite heavy use of abstract words in his speech. For example, he called a zebra crossing a 'safety plan' and medical notes 'a list of fictions' (*see* Table 7.1). One way of explaining this is to argue that abstract and concrete words are encoded differently in the semantic system and therefore are vulnerable to different effects following brain damage.

Unfortunately, a semantic problem will impair reading just as much as speech comprehension, since the person is unable to access meaning even from the written word. However, understanding of nonverbal modalities may be preserved, and we can help these people by accompanying our speech with gestures, pointing and even drawings.

Problems with sentences

In Table 7.1 Speaker 2 showed that dysphasia may leave single-word speech relatively intact but may severely disrupt the production of sentences. There are different types of sentence deficit in dysphasia (Berndt, 1991) with some people's difficulties confined to grammatical words and endings. This makes their speech 'telegrammatic', as is seen in the following extract:

> Speaker A: 'Valerie is big. Fat round hip. She quite tall. She work British Telecom. She always borrow pattern and not bring back'.

This is a very pure example of the problem; indeed we can 'correct' this person's language simply by restoring the grammatical words and endings; e.g. 'She **is** always borrow**ing** patterns and not br**inging them** back.'

Why are the grammatical elements omitted? This speaker had a problem pronouncing words, her speech was hesitant and contained a lot of struggling. It is possible therefore that she deliberately left out the grammatical words and inflections, in order to reduce the effort of talking. This would be sensible, since her meaning is clear despite the omission. However, this person also left out the grammatical words in her writing and found them difficult to read and understand, which suggested that she had a more general problem with them.

One factor which makes grammatical words difficult is their intangible meaning. Most of us could explain the meaning of main nouns and verbs, such as 'table' and 'walk', but would struggle with grammatical words like 'is' or 'of'. Indeed, these words are defined more by their use in sentences than in isolation. This may be precisely the problem for dysphasic people. Without a clear and concrete meaning, these words may be particularly vulnerable in certain cases of brain damage.

The above example shows that quite a lot of meaning may be communicated despite a problem with grammatical words. Of course, it is difficult for these speakers to formulate 'correct' questions or verb tense. However, dysphasic people often have clever strategies for overcoming these problems:

> They may use a statement with rising intonation to convey a question: 'New car?'

Dysphasic people also use explicit 'time signals' in place of tense: 'Last Saturday, visit sister.'

Given that meaning can be conveyed so successfully, it is often inappropriate to expect aphasic people to produce grammatically correct output. This point is eloquently made by Chris Ireland, who is herself a person with aphasia (Ireland & Black, 1992).

'If the person is somebody with aphasia, that person should say if they don't understand, like you would anyone else. That's respect. But people who correct you in the middle of you speaking, they make me furious. They shut you up. If people knew what I am trying to say well enough to correct, why bother? What are they doing putting on a model of perfect standard language? None of us grammatic correct all the time. People do not talk like that, so why correct people with aphasia?'

In line with this, therapy with such speakers may not aim to produce 'perfect' language – rather to promote strategies for conveying meaning despite the problems.

Sentence disorders in dysphasia can be more extensive. Many people have a problem composing word order (Saffran *et al.*, 1980). Here speech may be reduced to single words, or the person may try to string words together with anomalous results:

Speaker B: 'in the pet shop one woman and a cat is buying the man and paying the money the till.' (Description of a woman selling a cat to a man; Marshall *et al.*, 1997.)

The above speaker is interesting since many of the grammatical words which were difficult for speaker A are retained. Dissociations like this have encouraged the view that producing sentences involves at least two stages (Garrett, 1988). One stage composes the word order, and this has apparently failed for speaker B. The other applied the grammatical words and endings, and this has broken down in speaker A.

Problems with word order are very communicatively damaging (at least for English speakers), since this is our main device for expressing meaning. Thus, in Speaker B's sentence we can guess that someone is buying a cat in a pet shop, but have no means of knowing whether the man or woman is the purchaser. Because of the communicative implications clinicians have tried to develop new therapies to promote word order skills in aphasia.

Some sentence problems in aphasia are a product of other difficulties. For example, a severe word finding problem will affect sentence formulation. Many dysphasic people have a particular word finding difficulty with verbs (Miceli *et al.*, 1984; Berndt *et al.*, 1997a and b as shown by Speaker 2 in Table 7.1). Verbs play a very important role in sentences; and indeed, without them sentence production is impossible. Therefore this has also been a focus in recent aphasia therapies (Mitchum & Berndt, 1994).

Problems with sentence comprehension

There are many dysphasic people who understand single words well but have a variety of sentence comprehension problems. Some people's comprehension is affected by sentence length, and they might understand a sentence with just two key words, such as 'the *rotweiler* is *barking*', but not one with three key words, e.g. 'the *rotweiler* is *barking* at the *postman*'. This problem may be related to an impairment in short term or working memory that limits the amount of verbal information which can be retained. However, some commentators have disputed this and argue that memory plays only a very minor role in sentence comprehension (Gathercole & Baddeley, 1993).

Many people with dysphasia apparently can hold onto sentences, but still cannot understand them. Identifying such difficulties requires subtle testing. One approach is to ask the person to match a spoken sentence to a picture. By carefully controlling the sentences and the pictures, we can gather insights into what aspects of language are understood by the person and what are not.

For example, the therapist might show the dysphasic person four pictures of the following situations: boy kicking a ball; girl kicking a ball; boy holding a ball; boy kicking a cat.

The therapist then then asks the person to show her one picture by saying, 'Show me the boy kicking the ball.'

Let's imagine that the person succeeds which indicates that he or she understood all the key words, since missing just one could result in the wrong selection. If this is supported by other successes at this level, we can be reasonably confident that this client can process and retain at least three items of information.

The therapist now introduces a new set of stimuli by showing these pictures: man kissing a woman; woman kissing a man; man carrying a woman; man kissing a baby.

Her instruction to the client is: 'Show me: the man kissing the woman.'

Now the person is unsure and rapidly rejects the last two pictures but cannot choose between the first two. Furthermore, he or she displays the same pattern with several other 'reversible' sentences involving two people. It seems that the client is unable to interpret word order. He or she knows that some kissing is taking place between a man and a woman but cannot determine who is kissing whom. This is a fairly common problem in aphasia (Schwartz *et al.*, 1980; Black *et al.*, 1992) and has been related to word order problems in production (i.e. this client would probably also find it very difficult to describe these pictures).

Other dysphasic people can understand simple word order well, but not complex forms like passives ('the man was kissed by the woman') and sentences with embedded clauses. For example, on hearing the following sentence, the person may be unsure about who is the Scot: 'The man who came from Scotland kissed the woman.' Part of the difficulty here may relate to the comprehension of grammatical words and endings (you will remember that these can be a problem in production). As a result, clinicians often advise relatives and friends to avoid structures which make heavy use of these elements.

Jargon dysphasia

In jargon dysphasia 'normal' language has apparently been replaced by a startling new type of speech containing novel structures and made-up words (*see* Speaker 3, Table 7.1). Usually comprehension is severely impaired (Butterworth, 1985). Perhaps most puzzling is the fact that people with jargon aphasia seem unaware that their speech is at all peculiar and often become very angry when relatives and friends fail to understand them, and reject the offer of speech and language therapy. Some researchers have asked people with jargon aphasia to listen to tape recordings of their speech. Interestingly, these individuals maintained that nothing was wrong, although they did acknowledge their errors when they were spoken by another person (Kinsbourne & Warrington, 1964).

Jargon dysphasia is very poorly understood. First, we do not know why jargon speakers cannot detect their own errors. One theory suggests that self-monitoring has broken down because of the auditory comprehension deficit. In effect, this argues that the person can no longer hear themselves speak. However, the existence of jargon speakers with quite good comprehension has challenged this view (Maher *et al.*, 1994). Alternatively, these people may be denying their speech deficit in order to preserve a normal self-image (Weinstein, 1981; Prigatano & Weinstein, 1996). However, if this was the case we would expect error awareness to be obliterated, whereas, in fact, it is often patchy. For example, we have worked with a man who notices his errors in repetition, but not in naming (Marshall *et al.*, submitted) and another woman who notices her errors in writing but not speech (Robson *et al.*, in press). We are still at a loss to explain the monitoring failure in jargon and can only say that the specialized processes which detect errors in speech have for some reason failed and that the reason for that failure probably varies from person to person.

Another puzzling feature of jargon is the presence of neologisms, or novel words that seem to be entirely random. However, research has shown that they are not. Firstly, they tend to follow a pause or delay in the speech stream. Secondly, they usually replace content word vocabulary, such as main nouns and verbs. Thirdly, neologisms often retain grammatical endings, for example, one neologistic speaker said 'cherching' (for chasing) and 'rokes' (for robes) (Ellis *et al.*, 1983). Finally, neologisms often sound similar to one another.

Butterworth (1979, 1985) used such evidence to argue that neologisms are produced in response to a word finding deficit. This is what happens: first, the dysphasic person hunts for the word he wants, hence the delay. This is unsuccessful, so he generates a nonsense word to fill its place. The process which attaches grammatical endings is still functioning, so, as a result, his neologisms are usually inflected. Once produced, neologisms are held in an internal memory, or store, which explains why subsequent neologisms often sound like the first one.

We have recently conducted an extensive investigation of the neologisms produced by one aphasic speaker. On first inspection, these neologisms seemed to be completely unrelated to any target and were virtually impossible to understand. However, when we transcribed and analysed the utterances, we found that they did contain at least some of the sounds of the target word, and more so than would be expected by chance. Like Butterworth, we concluded that this speaker was attempting to retrieve target words, but was encountering word finding problems. Despite these problems, he was accessing some of the target sounds. These were then combined with more randomly activated sounds in order to construct a neologism (Robson *et al.*, in preparation).

Theories of neologism production leave many questions unanswered such as why people with jargon aphasia produce neologisms, rather than remain silent? It may be that they do not know that they are making errors, as discussed above. Alternatively, they may know, but decide to produce them anyway. In other words, they may prefer to make mistakes than be rendered speechless.

Problems with reading and writing

Reading and writing in aphasia are just as vulnerable as speech, and the pattern of strengths and weaknesses across the modalities can vary considerably. Someone with little or no speech may preserve some useful writing, while someone with very poor auditory comprehension may still be able to read (assuming, of course, that they were pre-morbidly literate). Disorders of reading and writing following neurological damage are called respectively dyslexia and dysgraphia. Although these are typically part of the dysphasic complex, they can occur in isolation. Perhaps most surprisingly, they can also dissociate. In other words, we occasionally encounter people who can write but not read and vice versa.

Investigations of reading aim to find out what types of words and sentences can still be read, and what use the person is able to make of this skill. Obviously, it is very important to test reading comprehension, especially as some people who have had strokes can read words aloud without understanding them. To do this, clinicians may ask the person to match words to pictures or to answer questions about the meanings of words. Therapists also try to find out how the person used reading and writing before their stroke, since this varies a lot in the general population (Parr, 1992). This information is crucial when planning therapy, e.g. there is no point in trying to help a person write letters, if he or she never corresponded before suffering the stroke.

Research has shown that certain classes of words can cause particular difficulties following strokes, depending on the type of disorder (Ellis, 1993). For example, some people become heavily dependent on letter to sound correspondences in their reading, a problem called Surface Dyslexia (Patterson, Marshall and Coltheart, 1985). Thus, they can read regular words like 'boat', but not irregular ones like 'yacht'. When faced with the irregular items, they may try to sound them out from their letters, i.e. by saying 'yakt' or may just look totally puzzled and deny that the word exists.

Another criteria is the meaning of the word. Many dyslexic people cannot read abstract words like 'idea' and 'democracy', but cope reasonably with concrete ones like 'pram' and 'television'. These subjects may also fail with grammatical words, like 'is' and 'of', despite the fact that these words are very common and usually very short. This latter problem can make the reading of sentences difficult. People who show these signs are thought to have a problem in their semantic system, which makes the reading of all words without concrete meanings very difficult.

A third factor which affects reading for many people is how frequently the word is used. For example, very common words, like 'car', may be read, whereas uncommon ones like 'ant' may not be. Clinicians will try to tease out these reading patterns in their clients, partly because the patterns provide clues about what aspects of language are still functioning but also because they are helpful in planning therapy and advising family and friends. Thus, if a person has a particular difficulty with irregular words, the therapist can advise carers to avoid them.

Writing disorders are common in aphasia. Of course, many dysphasic people have to write with their non-preferred hand, because of a hemiplegia. However, this is not the primary cause of the writing deficit, contrary to the belief of many relatives and friends. This can be demonstrated by asking the person to spell a word by using letter tiles. If he or she still has a problem, we can be sure that the dysgraphia is not simply due to difficulties with the pen. It seems that the person can no longer access information about how words should be spelt.

There are different levels and types of writing disorders in aphasia. In some cases writing may be entirely impossible. Others can still write very familiar words and phrases, such as their own name and possibly parts of their address, but little else. When writing is more extensive, similar patterns to those outlined above may emerge. For example, common or regularly spelt words may be achieved, while irregular or abstract words may be very difficult. Some of the speech patterns described can also appear in writing. Thus, writing may lack sentence structure or may consist of jargon. Dysphasic people who still write with their preferred hand can often execute a perfect signature, regardless of the general status of their writing, probably because the signature is a learnt movement pattern, rather than a genuine literary act.

Articulatory dyspraxia

Some speech problems following stroke are due to dyspraxia, or apraxia, which is the inability to carry out purposeful, willed movement, although the same movements can be performed spontaneously. For example, the person may be unable to vocalize to command but will shout out spontaneously if he drops his coffee or stubs his toe. Dyspraxia is not due to muscle weakness or paralysis. There are many different manifestations of this disorder, such as limb dyspraxia, dressing dyspraxia, and the dyspraxia which affects speech, articulatory dyspraxia.

Someone with a pure articulatory dyspraxia shows the following signs:

- Language is intact, and therefore reading and comprehension are preserved. The person should also be able to write, providing there is no associated limb dyspraxia.
- There is no facial weakness. The mouth does not droop to one side, and spontaneous facial movements, such as smiling and grimacing, are normal (although there may be difficulty in carrying out these movements to request). Most importantly, eating and drinking, which use the same muscles as speech, are accomplished effortlessly.

Despite the absence of facial paralysis, the person may experience extreme problems whenever speech is attempted. Efforts to talk are accompanied by groping and struggle behaviours, as the person tries to make his or her tongue and lips carry out the desired movements. This client may also attempt to correct pronunciation errors, which shows that he or she has a good idea about what the word should sound like. All tasks involving speech should be affected. Therefore, if the person can repeat or read aloud but not talk spontaneously, the problem is probably not dyspraxia.

Dyspraxia varies in severity. In its most extreme form speech may be impossible, whereas other individuals preserve a single word or phrase, which appears whenever speech is attempted (Blanken *et al.*, 1989; Code, 1994). These stereotyped utterances may be connected with the person's former lifestyle. For example, the neurologist Hughlings Jackson described a patient who was a clerk and could only say 'list complete' (Lebrun, 1986). However, many recurrent utterances do not have a personal connection. Often the one word that can still be said is an expletive, possibly because this vocabulary is more 'automatic' and therefore relatively untouched by a disorder that affects propositional or purposeful speech.

Milder dyspraxias permit more speech, although with considerable struggle and delay. They profoundly alter the way a person sounds. For example, any regional accent will probably be reduced, and the person may sound much younger or even rather aggressive. The rhythm, or prosody, of the speech will be severely disrupted. Pronunciation errors will be common and will fluctuate a great deal. For example, a dyspraxic person trying to say 'splash', might say 'spash', then 'stash', and then 'suckerplash'. This last example illustrates another common feature, namely errors of complication.

One condition which may accompany dyspraxia is known as foreign accent syndrome. As the term suggests, people with this syndrome seem to have acquired a novel accent, i.e. the person may sound Italian or French. Investigations suggest that the impression of foreignness arises from a number of distortions in the person's speech. For example, consonants and vowels are mispronounced, and stress and prosody may be disrupted (Ardila *et al.*, 1988; Berthier *et al.*, 1991). Foreign accent syndrome can be very distressing, as it profoundly affects a person's self-image and can lead to embarrassing misunderstandings. However, not all individuals regret the disorder. One person, known to the author, was very anxious that the therapist should *not* remove his acquired French accent, as it gave him a new cachet with girl friends.

Dyspraxia need not occur in isolation, indeed it quite frequently accompanies dysphasia. This can create problems of diagnosis, since the clinician must determine whether symptoms are due to the language disorder or to the dyspraxia. It is particularly difficult to isolate dyspraxic problems from phonological problems, especially if the client has very little speech. One means of doing this is to ask the person to make judgements about the sounds of words. For example, when showing the person three pictures – a house, a cat and a hat – the clinician asks the client to indicate which two pictures have rhyming names, without saying the words aloud. If the client can do this, he or she must be able to access the phonologies of the pictured words. We can therefore be more confident in attributing the speech problems to dyspraxia. Dual disorders also generate management problems, and the clinician has to decide whether to treat the dysphasia or the dyspraxia.

Dysarthria

Dysarthria is a speech impairment arising from paralysed or un-coordinated muscles, specifically in the lips, tongue, soft palate and larynx. When dysarthria is very severe, rendering speech uninterpretable, it is termed *anarthria*. In strokes, dysarthria occurs because the nerve supply to the speech muscles has been damaged. In pure dysarthria the person's language is unaffected, comprehension is normal, and he or she will be able to read and write. Depending on manual skills, the person will also be able to make good use of computers and other communication aids.

Single strokes rarely lead to dysarthria, except for strokes affecting the brain stem, as this is where the nerves directly supplying the speech muscles originate. Otherwise, persistent dysarthrias tend to follow multiple strokes because speech movement is controlled by cortical areas on both sides of the brain and is therefore only disrupted by bilateral damage.

Unlike dyspraxia, dysarthria is signalled by obvious muscle weakness or paralysis and an altered appearance of the face. The mouth may hang open, and there may be drooping of the lips and a flaccidity in the cheeks. Another sign is persistent drooling of saliva. Speech is slurred, indistinct and frequently hypernasal, because palatal involvement allows air to escape through the nose. Volume is usually reduced, because of poor breath support and weakness in the larynx. In spastic dysarthrias, where muscle tone is abnormally elevated, speech may feature explosive bursts, as the person struggles to initiate voice. Speech errors are fairly consistent with vowel sounds, which are made with an open mouth, often the least affected. Indeed, in severe dysarthria these may be the only sounds that can be achieved.

The muscle disorder will be evident in all activities involving the mouth. Therefore, dysphagia, or a disorder in eating and drinking, is to be anticipated. For example, tongue weakness results in an inability to move food round the mouth during chewing, or to collect it and move it back in preparation for the swallow. Alternatively, or additionally, the swallow reflex may be weakened or delayed. As a result, food may pass to the back of the mouth and into the trachea before the swallow is triggered. Alarmingly, a number of people with dysphagia also have a weakened cough, which means that they cannot expel food once it has dropped into the trachea. Dysphagia therefore requires urgent management, not only for nutritional reasons, but also because it leads to chest infections, as food passes into the lungs.

As with dyspraxia, dysarthria may be accompanied by other neurological impairments, particularly when the person has had more than one stroke. For example, there may be a secondary language disorder or cognitive impairment. This rarely impedes diagnosis, as dysarthria is relatively easy to identify; however, it will profoundly affect management, since the person may be unable to respond to therapy or apply problem solving strategies.

Acknowledgements

This chapter was prepared while the author was supported by MRC Grant Number: G9231810N.

References

Ardila, A., Rosselli, M. & Ardila, O. (1988) Foreign accent syndrome: an aphasic epiphenomenon. *Aphasiology* **2**, 493–9.

Beaton, A., Guest, J. & Ved, R. (1997) Semantic errors of naming, reading, writing and drawing following left hemisphere infarction. *Cognitive Neuropsychology* **14**, 459–78.

Berndt, R. (1991) Sentence processing in aphasia. In *Acquired Aphasia* (M.T. Sarno, ed.). Academic Press, New York.

Berndt, R., Mitchum, C., Haendiges, A. & Sandson, J. (1997a) Verb retrieval in aphasia: 1, Characterising single word impairments. *Brain and Language* **56**, 68–107.

Berndt, R., Haendiges, A., Mitchum, C. & Sandson, J. (1997b) Verb retrieval in aphasia: 2, Relationship to sentence processing. *Brain and Language* **56**, 107–29.

Berthier, M., Ruiz, A., Massone, M., Starkstein, S. & Leiguarda, R. (1991) Foreign accent syndrome: behavioural and anatomical findings in recovered and non-recovered patients. *Aphasiology* **5**, 129–47.

Best, W. (1995) A reverse length effect in dysphasic naming: when elephant is easier than ant. *Cortex* **31**, 637–53.

Black, M., Nickels, L. & Byng, S. (1992) Patterns of sentence processing deficit: processing simple sentences can be a complex matter. *Journal of Neurolinguistics* **6**, 79–101.

Blanken, G., de Langen, E., Dittmann, J. & Wallesch, C. (1989) Implications of preserved written language abilities for the functional basis of speech automatisms (recurring utterances): A single case study. *Cognitive Neuropsychology* **6**, 211–49.

Bonita, R. & Anderson, A. (1983) Speech and language disorders after stroke: an epidemiological study. *New Zealand Speech and Language Therapy Journal* **38**, 2–9.

Butterworth, B. (1979) Hesitation and the production of verbal paraphasis and neologisms in jargon aphasia. *Brain and Language* **8**, 133–61.

Butterworth, B. (1985) Jargon aphasia: processes and strategies. In *Current Perspectives in Dysphasia* (S. Newman and R. Epstein, eds). Churchill Livingstone, Edinburgh.

Code, C. (1994) Speech automatism production in aphasia. *Journal of Neurolinguistics* **8**, 135–48.

Coltheart, M., Patterson, K. & Marshall, J. (1980) *Deep Dyslexia.* Routledge and Kegan Paul, London.

Damasio, H. (1991) Neuroanatomical correlates of the aphasias. In *Acquired Aphasia* (M.T. Sarno, ed.). Academic Press, New York.

Ellis, A. (1993) *Reading, Writing and Dyslexia: A Cognitive Analysis* (second edition). Lawrence Erlbaum, London.

Ellis, A., Miller, D. & Sin, G. (1983) Wernicke's aphasia and normal language processing: a case study in cognitive neuropsychology. *Cognition* **15**, 110–45.

Ellis, A. & Young, A. (1996) *Human Cognitive Neuropsychology* (second edition). Lawrence Erlbaum, Hove.

Franklin, S. (1989) Dissociations in auditory word comprehension: evidence from nine fluent aphasic patients. *Aphasiology* **3**, 189–207.

Franklin, S., Howard, D. & Patterson, K. (1994) Abstract word meaning deafness. *Cognitive Neuropsychology* **11**, 1–34.

Franklin, S., Howard, D. & Patterson, K. (1995) Abstract word anomia. *Cognitive Neuropsychology* **12**, 549–66.

Garrett, M. (1988) Processes in language production. In *Linguistics: The Cambridge Survey* 3 (F.J. Newmeyer, ed.). Cambridge University Press, Cambridge.

Gathercole, S. & Baddeley, A. (1993) *Working Memory and Language.* Lawrence Erlbaum, Hove.

Howard, D. & Orchard-Lisle, V. (1984) On the origin of semantic errors in naming: evidence from the case of a global aphasic. *Cognitive Neuropsychology* **1**, 163–90.

Howard, D., Patterson, K., Franklin, S., Morton, J. & Orchard-Lisle, V. (1984) Variability and consistency in picture naming in aphasic patients. In *Advances in Neurology, 42; Progress in aphasiology* (F.C. Rose, ed.). Raven Press, New York.

Hillis, A., Rapp, B., Romani, C. & Caramazza, A. (1990) A selective impairment of semantics in lexical processing. *Cognitive Neuropsychology* **7**, 191–243.

Ireland, C. & Black, M. (1992) Living with aphasia: the insight story. *UCL Working Papers in Linguistics* **4**. University College, London.

Kay, J. & Ellis, A. (1987) A cognitive neuropsychological case study of anomia: implications for psychological models of word retrieval. *Brain* **110**, 613–29.

Kay, J., Lesser, R. & Coltheart, M. (1992) *Psycholinguistic Assessment of Language Processing in Aphasia.* Lawrence Erlbaum, Hillsdale, New Jersey.

Kinsbourne, M. & Warrington, E. (1963) Jargon aphasia. *Neuropsychologia* **1**, 27–37.

Lebrun, Y. (1986) Aphasia with recurrent utterance: a review. *British Journal of Disorders of Communication* **21**, 3–10.

Lucchelli, F. & De Renzi, E. (1992) Proper name anomia. *Cortex* **28**, 221–30.

Marshall, J., Robson, J., Pring, T. & Chiat, S. (1998) Why does monitoring fail in jargon aphasia: comprehension, judgement and therapy evidence. *Brain and Language* **63**, 79–107.

Marshall, J., Pring, T., Chiat, S. & Robson, J. (1996) Calling a salad a federation: an investigation of semantic jargon, part 1: nouns. *Journal of Neurolinguistics* **9**, 237–50.

Marshall, J., Chiat, S., Robson, J. & Pring, T. (1996) Calling a salad a federation: an investigation of semantic jargon, part 2: verbs. *Journal of Neurolinguistics* **9**, 251–60.

Marshall, J., Chiat, S. & Pring, T. (1997) An impairment in processing verbs' thematic roles: a therapy study. *Aphasiology* **11**, 855–76.

Maher, L., Gonzalez Rothi, L. & Heilman, K. (1994) Lack of error awareness in an aphasic patient with relatively preserved auditory comprehension. *Brain and Language* **46**, 402–18.

Miceli, G., Silveri, M., Villa, G. & Caramazza, A. (1984) On the basis of the agrammatic's difficulty in producing main verbs. *Cortex* **20**, 207–20.

Mitchum, C. & Berndt, R. (1994) Verb retrieval and sentence construction: Effects of targeted intervention. In *Cognitive Neuropsychology and Cognitive Rehabilitation* (G.W. Humphreys & J. Riddoch, eds). Lawrence Erlbaum, Hove.

Parr, S. (1992) Everyday reading and writing practices of normal adults: implications for aphasia assessment. *Aphasiology* **6**, 273–85.

Patterson, K., Marshall, J. & Coltheart, M. (eds) (1985) *Surface Dyslexia*. Laurence Erlbaum, London.

Prigatano, G. & Weinstein, E. (1996) Edwin A. Weinstein's contributions to neuropsychological rehabilitation. *Neuropsychological Rehabilitation* **6**, 305–26.

Robson, J., Pring, T., Marshall, J., Morrison, S. & Chiat S. (1998) Written communication in undifferentiated jargon aphasia: a therapy study. *International Journal of Language and Communication Disorders* **33**, 305–28.

Saffran, E., Schwartz, M. & Marin, O. (1980) The word order problem in agrammatism. 2: production. *Brain and Language* **10**, 263–80.

Schwartz, M., Saffran, E. & Marin, O. (1980) The word order problem in agrammatism. 1: comprehension. *Brain and Language* **10**, 249–62.

Weinstein, E. (1981) Behavioural aspects of jargon aphasia. In *Jargonaphasia* (J. Brown, ed.). Academic Press, New York.

Chapter 8

The Treatment of Speech and Language Disorders Following Stroke

Jane Marshall

Treatment of aphasia

Aphasia therapy is a complex process which, ideally, takes place over a long period of time. It incorporates many aims, such as:

- To alleviate the language disorder.
- To help the person compensate for the language disorder.
- To help those in contact with the dysphasic person understand the language disorder and to offer methods for improving communication at home.
- To help the person (and his or her family) deal with the psychological and social consequences of aphasia.

Aphasia therapy rarely tackles all these aims at once. Instead, the focus changes and develops over time. For example, immediately after the stroke, the therapist may concentrate on supporting the patient and his or her family. Later on, specific language work might be started and this, in turn, may incorporate compensatory work. The main participants in aphasia therapy are the dysphasic person and the speech and language therapist. The patient's family and friends should also be involved and possibly volunteers and assistants.

This section covers the first three aims of aphasia therapy as well as some general service issues which are the subject of current debate.

Alleviating the language disorder

Much aphasia therapy aims to improve damaged language skills. Often the first question is which skill or skills to concentrate on, since language problems are generally multiple. For example, the person may have difficulties with word finding, reading and writing, so the therapist will try to identify which problem is most affecting communication. Thus in our example, the aphasic person may report that the word finding problem is paramount, as it disrupts conversation, and that reading and writing are less of a priority. The therapist will, therefore, make this the initial focus of therapy. Of course, priorities can change over time, as impairments evolve and different needs emerge.

Once a focus for therapy has been determined, the therapist will carry out an assessment which aims to uncover the nature of the impairment in that area and any residual skills that could help the patient overcome, or compensate for, the problem. The findings of this assessment are used to generate a 'therapy hypothesis' which guides the selection and administration of the treatment tasks (Jones & Byng, 1988).

I shall illustrate this process through an example of naming therapy (Marshall, 1989; Marshall *et al.*, 1990). The subject in this study, RS, had a severe naming problem. For example, when shown 25 pictures of common objects he could name only 8. More importantly, this anomia profoundly disrupted conversation, partly because he had few strategies for coping with the problem. Accordingly, we decided to tackle it in therapy.

Assessment showed that RS had some important skills. His comprehension was excellent, both in conversation and in testing: i.e. he could match a spoken word to one of five pictures very reliably, despite the fact that the pictures included items which were very closely related to the target. He could also judge the names of pictures. For example, if I showed him a picture of a fly and asked 'is this a spider', he would reply correctly. This showed that RS still had a good idea about the meaning of words. In other words, his semantic system, at least for concrete items, was intact.

Next I was interested in whether RS still knew about the sounds of words (or their phonologies). Here the most useful clue came from his reading. RS could read any word aloud, regardless of its length, spelling or meaning. It seemed that words' phonologies were still in his system and that he could produce them, provided he was given the written word as a cue.

The last question was whether RS could write names. If he could, they would provide an obvious strategy for his problem. Unfortunately, assessment showed that his written naming was no better than spoken. Furthermore, he could only write the name of a picture once he had said it.

These assessments generated a number of therapy hypotheses. It seemed that RS's naming problem was not due to a deficit either in his semantic system or in the phonological store. I had to infer that his problem lay in the connections between the two. In other words, when trying to name something, RS had a good idea about the meaning of the required word, but could no longer access its sound, unless he was given the written word as a cue.

Clearly therapy should try to help RS reconnect the meanings of words with their sounds. To do this I used tasks which exploited his two main skills, namely his good comprehension and reading. In one task, he was shown a picture of a TV alongside five written words consisting of the target and four related items: a radio, a television, a record player, a video, a camera.

RS was required to find the correct word and read it aloud. Thus, he had to access both the meaning and the sound of the target word. RS was also invited to 'brainstorm' ideas related to the target picture. Thus, for TV, he might generate: 'aerial', *Radio Times* and 'Eastenders' (these were often conveyed through non-verbal means, such as drawing, miming or even singing the signature tune). This element of the therapy encouraged him to circumlocute more – or communicate information about the meaning of the word. Two benefits from this were envis-aged: firstly, by circumlocuting he might cue himself to name the object; secondly, he could use this as a strategy in conversation, to help people guess his targets.

Only three hours were spent on this therapy, but there were some promising gains. RS could now name 20 out of 25 of the items which he had practised in therapy, and he maintained this score after a month's break. There was another encouraging sign. I asked RS to name 12 items which were related to words used in therapy, although not specifically worked on. He scored 11 out of 12, indicating that the treatment may have benefited words that were similar in meaning to the therapy items. However, untreated items which were unrelated to the therapy items showed no change, indicating that his naming had not generally improved.

Whether the therapy had eased conversation was much more difficult to assess. However, there were some hints. After therapy, RS showed a novel capacity for overcoming anomic blocks, either by eventually reaching his target or through compensating techniques such as providing related alternatives or using gesture. Below are some examples taken from a conversation about his business:

Therapist: 'What will you do with the capital?'
RS: 'Put it into the ... one in the ... what's name ... bank.'

RS: 'Er one chap has come up with a ... er ... fee' (target offer).

Therapist: 'What's happening to the staff?'
RS: 'Er ... er ... (waves) goodbye, goodbye.'

This is quite a good example of what can be achieved by naming therapy. A number of studies show that we can help people improve their production of treated words (Nettleton & Lesser, 1991; Nickels & Best, 1996). Furthermore, these effects can show excellent maintenance (Pring *et al.*, 1990). Some naming studies also show generalization to words which are semantically related to those which have been worked on, and a few report better naming of all words fol-lowing therapy (Nickels & Best, 1996; Jones, 1989). It seems that therapy can train vocabulary, and we can be reasonably confident that this training will 'stick'. While not solving the problem, this can be useful if the vocabulary is carefully chosen for its relevance to the patient. However, such training need not be the only gain from therapy. More importantly we can promote strategies for coping with anomia. Thus, RS was more able to circumlocute the gesture after therapy – and this was with all words, not just those which had featured in treatment.

Not all language therapy focuses on naming. Treatments have also been devised to improve comprehension (Behrmann & Lieberthal, 1989), reading (De Partz, 1986; Scott & Byng, 1989) and writing (Behrmann, 1987). There have also been several accounts of therapies for sentence production and comprehension (Jones, 1986; Byng, 1988; and see Marshall, 1995, for review), as described in the following study (Marshall *et al.*, 1997).

The subject of this study, PB, produced speech which was superficially grammatical – e.g. it had syntactic structure and contained grammatical words and endings (Marshall *et al.*, 1997). Despite this, PB was often very difficult to understand, as shown in this conversation sample:

PB: 'The garage is ringing M to say the car is bringing the truck ... no.'
JM: 'So the garage rang M?'
PB: 'No, M rang the garage ... could it be possible ... bring the car, a truck.'
(Target: Martin rang the garage to ask them to pick up his car with a truck.)

Thus, PB was poor at expressing meaning, partly because he often used the wrong verb, such as 'bring'. Even when the verb was correct, PB displayed a secondary problem with word order, and in the sample he initially misorders the nouns around 'ring'.

PB's problems were not confined to production: he also found it difficult to comprehend word order. For example, if he heard the sentence 'The man carries the woman', he might match it to a picture of a woman carrying a man. Some single verbs were also difficult for him to understand, and verbs expressing change of possession (like 'buy'/'sell' and 'lend'/'borrow') were the most problematic.

I hypothesized that therapy should focus on the meaning expressed by verbs and sentences. If successful, this should benefit both production and comprehension. The tasks exploited change of possession verbs. In the first phase PB was required to read and understand sentences containing these verbs. These were colour coded so that the person receiving the object was marked in red: e.g. John gave a jumper to *Bob*.

PB was given a number of picture cards representing the people and objects. For each written sentence, he was asked to find the relevant cards and use them to represent the described event. In order to capture the change of possession, he was required to move the object card in the appropriate direction between the two people. Questions and discussed further emphasized the meaning of the sentence and how it related to word order. For example, the therapist might ask: 'who ends up with the jumper?' and point out that this person is expressed after the verb.

As PB became proficient in this task, new stages were introduced. First of all, the colour coding was eliminated; then alternative sentence forms were used: e.g. John gave Bob a jumper.

Finally the tasks moved on to production, as illustrated in Fig. 8.1. Here PB was

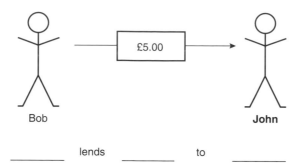

Fig. 8.1 A change of possession event. The bold word would actually be in red, and indicates the recipient of the action.

given a drawing showing a change of possession event. This was colour coded so that the recipient was marked in red. Below the picture was a colour coded sentence frame. PB had to fill in the missing nouns. As before, discussion drew his attention to the direction of the event and how this related to the position of the nouns. Therapy spanned 12 sessions with intervening homework.

Following therapy, PB's production of change of possession sentences improved, as measured by picture description and a story retelling task. His comprehension of the treated type of verb also improved. Encouragingly the gain generalized to verbs which had not been specifically worked on. For example, 'sell' was not a treated verb, but PB was still able to use it better after therapy, as illustrated in the following sample:

'Mary went to the house to the neighbour ... to buy the car off the neighbour ... no ... no, no, sell the ... Mary is selling the car to the neighbour.'

This comparatively short programme of therapy enabled PB to express and comprehend change of possession verbs more effectively. As these had been particularly problematic prior to therapy, this was a valuable result. For example, PB was now much more able to discuss the selling of his house, which was an issue that greatly preoccupied him at the time of the therapy programme.

These brief examples illustrate some of the general features of this type of treatment. Firstly, there is a hypothesis about what aspects of language processing are either impaired or intact. Therapy is developed in the light of this hypothesis. Thus, with RS, I hypothesized that naming was failing because of a break-down in the links between semantics and phonology. Therapy aimed to restore those links partly by exploiting RS's strengths, i.e. in reading aloud and making judgements about word meanings.

Usually, the therapy programme is hierarchical, or tasks become progressively more difficult. An example of this was the elimination of colour coding from PB's materials and the introduction of alternative syntactic forms. There is also considerable discussion during therapy about the purpose and aims of the task, and about how the person is doing. Most therapists regard this feedback as crucial to the treatment (Byng & Jones, 1993), since it helps the person to develop insights about the nature of the problem and how to overcome it. These interactions require considerable therapeutic skill. They demand a firm grasp of the aims of therapy, as well as the ability to observe the patient very closely and interpret his or her performance. Such observations may also lead to modifications of the therapy task, e.g. in response to persistent failure.

This summary shows that, like all therapy, treatment for language impairments is extremely complex, despite the fact that the tasks used are often very simple. It is therefore difficult for untrained volunteers and assistants to carry out the planning for this type of work, but they can very usefully supplement it. For example, volunteers and assistants often administer practice tasks outside the therapy sessions, and relatives can help with homework. These contributions increase the person's exposure to the target language area and may help him or her to generalize skills beyond the therapy setting.

Compensating for the language disorder

The above section described treatments which aim directly to lessen the language impairment. This section will deal with therapies which compensate for that impairment. Of course, in practice therapists often address the two aims at once. Thus, the naming therapy with RS aimed to alleviate his anomia *and* give him strategies for coping with the problem.

There are many reasons for conducting compensatory therapy. It reduces frustration and can offer methods of communication prior to the restoration of speech. Above all it promotes problem solving abilities. Given the chronic nature of dysphasia, these are essential for the person's long-term well-being.

Compensatory therapies take many forms. Much of the work fosters helpful strategies which enable the person to 'bypass' specific problems. An example of this would be the agrammatic speaker who uses time signals, like 'yesterday', to replace absent tense markers. These strategies may be developed independently by the patient, in which case the therapist's role is simply to encourage them One member of our aphasia therapy group made very effective use of tunes to communicate – for example, he sang 'I do love to be beside the sea-side' to convey that he was going on holiday. This strategy was promoted through a task in which the group had to think of tunes to communicate different messages. As this suggests, group therapy can provide an excellent forum for working on problem solving devices, since here clients can experiment with different ideas and learn from one another.

In some cases it may be necessary to alter or replace maladaptive strategies. For example, one dysphasic client discovered that he could still count, despite the fact that he was otherwise speechless. From then on every communication attempt was accompanied by counting, which was extremely misleading for his conversational partners. This behaviour was reduced by encouraging him to write instead of speak and by working through his family and friends. Relatives were advised to tell him honestly that the counting did not help and to offer him a pencil and paper whenever he tried to communicate.

Many compensatory therapies teach alternative channels of communications, such as gesture and drawing. While some dysphasic people turn to these methods automatically, others need instruction. This may be because a hemiplegia or limb dyspraxia makes gesturing and drawing difficult. Alternatively, it may be because the language impairment has also affected nonverbal symbols.

A number of clinicians teach Amer-Ind, which is the sign language of the American Indians (Skelly, 1979). Amer-Ind has the advantage of being easily understood, even by someone who is unfamiliar with the system. It is also possible to do most of the signs with only one hand, which is of course essential for those dysphasic people who have a hemiplegia. McIntosh and Dakin (1989) described how they used Amer-Ind in the rehabilitation of a dysphasic man. Signs were taught in small groups and in naturalistic contexts. For example, 'yes', 'no', 'drink', 'sugar' and 'milk' were introduced in a tea making session. The therapists used gestures rather than speech during these sessions, both in order to demonstrate the signs and to show that nonverbal communication was effective. Gradually the therapists built up the patient's signing vocabulary until he was able to convey quite complex messages. For example, in one session he recounted that he had seen a car with a speaking computer which had amazed his grandson. Without his signing system this man would have been unable to communicate, since, even eight months post-onset, his writing was poor and speech was limited to stereotyped phrases.

Drawing therapies promote another useful alternative to speech. Some tasks aim to improve the clarity of drawing in order to facilitate communication. Fawcus and Lawson (in press) asked their group members to draw different fruits and then highlighted the distinguishing features between the items. Lyon (1995) describes a 'magnifying glass' strategy. Here patients are encouraged to blow up important sections of their drawing to clarify them for the viewer. Once clarity is established, further work may be needed to encourage the communicative use of drawing. For example, one of our group members drew horses excellently but could not use this skill to tell us that he had been to a horse show over the weekend. Here assignments can be useful, in which the patient is required to communicate messages by using practised drawings. Lyon (1995) argues that drawings should only be used within a communicative context in therapy. His programme aims to develop interactive drawing where conversation is aided by both the aphasic and non-aphasic person using the medium.

A final word about compensatory therapies: some relatives and friends become anxious if compensatory techniques are suggested. One fear is that the use of signing or drawing may inhibit the return of speech. In fact, there is no evidence to support this view; and indeed one study suggests that gestures might facilitate, rather than hinder speech (Skelly *et al.*, 1974). Similarly, Cubelli (1995) describes a programme which aimed to improve a subject's drawing from memory, by encouraging him to illustrate the differentiating features between related objects. Following therapy this subject's spoken naming improved, particularly for items like animals and vegetables, which are mainly defined by their physical appearance.

Another fear is that the use of compensatory therapy signals a poor language prognosis. This fear is also often groundless. Clinicians advocate nonverbal strategies for many different reasons – principally to lessen frustration and to open a channel of communication before formal language skills return. The use of compensatory therapy is not a sign that the clinician has given up on speech.

Reducing the social consequences of aphasia

The preceding sections focused on therapies which aim to change the abilities and behaviours of the dysphasic person. This section describes approaches which aim to alter that person's environment, usually by changing the attitudes or behaviours of his or her family and friends. This approach represents an important philosophical shift. The problem of dysphasia is no longer seen as residing purely with the dysphasic person. It is also due to society's inability to accommodate people with different communication styles.

There is considerable evidence that aphasia is not only devastating for the person directly affected, but also for his or her 'carers'. For example, Kinsella and Duffy (1978) reported that aphasia was associated with a high incidence of depression and poor adjustment in the spouses of stroke patients. These effects may, in turn, impair the quality of communication at home and, possibly, the progress of therapy (Mulhall, 1978; Borenstein, 1993). Even when such negative effects are not present, the introduction of aphasia into a family requires new skills from everyone involved. We cannot assume that relatives and friends will automatically adapt their communication to meet the needs of the aphasic person. Yet without such adaptation, the person may become excluded from all former social ties.

A number of therapists have responded to the needs of families by running relative support groups. The issues covered by such groups can be wide ranging. The workshops described by Whitehead (1992) aimed to increase understanding about aphasia, develop problem solving skills, and offer opportunities for emotional support. Activities include explanatory sessions about particular aspects of aphasia, observation of therapy sessions, video and discussion. Although not formally evaluated, the groups seemed to promote greater insight amongst those attending and, thereby, improved interactions. In particular, they helped to overcome some relatives' previous opposition to total communication strategies.

Lesser and Algar (1995) also describe a therapy programme involving family members. As part of their therapy, they recorded conversations between the aphasic person and a 'caregiver'. These recordings were analysed, using Conversational Analysis, in order to determine what kinds of difficulties occurred in the interactions and how those difficulties were, or were not, resolved. These insights formed the basis of detailed advice sheets, which were given to the aphasic person and caregiver. So, for example, one caregiver might be advised to give the aphasic person more time to find target words. This advice was supported with a specific example from the recording, illustrating the successful use of the strategy. Re-assessment at the end of this intervention suggested that therapy brought about important changes in the interactions taking place between the aphasic people and their caregivers. For example, more successful repairs might be noted, or an increase in checking behaviours on the part of the caregiver.

Lesser and Algar's therapy mainly aimed to change the behaviours of caregivers, without necessarily improving the skills of the aphasic person. However, in other programmes dual aims may be adopted. Thus, McIntosh and Dakin (above) aimed to teach their patient signs and to encourage those round him to employ and elicit those signs. Similarly Lyon's drawing therapy (above) promoted drawing skills in the aphasic person and included a training element for conversational partners.

One of the most developed examples of therapy aiming to reduce the social consequences of aphasia takes place at the North York Aphasia Centre in Ontario (Kagan & Gailey, 1993). The centre makes extensive use of volunteers, who are trained in conversational techniques with aphasic people. These volunteers act as facilitators in conversational groups. The group programme does not set out to lessen the language impairments of the participants. Instead it aims to give people with aphasia renewed social access. The volunteers are compared to the aids used by people with physical disabilities. They promote communicative access, just as a wheelchair promotes physical access.

Efficacy of aphasia therapy

In recent years there has been considerable debate about whether aphasia therapy works. In part, this was stimulated by randomized controlled trials (RCTs) which showed either no improvement (Lincoln *et al.*, 1984) or that therapy was no more effective than volunteer support (Meikle *et al.*, 1979; David *et al.*, 1983).

Replies to these studies have argued that RCTs are not an appropriate method of evaluating aphasia therapy (Howard, 1986; Pring, 1986). This chapter has demonstrated that aphasia therapy is, in fact, an umbrella term covering a variety of interventions and techniques, all of which have different aims. In this context it is simply not sensible to ask whether aphasia therapy works. Instead we have to ask whether a particular intervention is successful in bringing about its desired aims. This question, by its very nature, cannot be answered by a large randomized trial. It can only be addressed through studies which evaluate one treatment with either an individual or a small group of subjects. We now have several studies of this kind which show positive outcomes (Byng & Coltheart, 1986; Pring *et al.*, 1990; Nickels *et al.*, 1991). Of course, these studies do not generalize about the entire dysphasic population, but they do confirm that therapy can achieve specific aims with particular people.

The therapy regime

Another topic of discussion is the optimum therapy regime. The issues here concern the best timing for intervention, whether therapy should be delivered individually or in groups and the frequency and duration of therapy.

Timing

Many clinicians believe that therapy should be introduced as early as possible after the stroke. This view is influenced by studies suggesting that therapy outcomes are adversely affected by delay (Sands *et al.*, 1969). One difficulty is that treatment effects may be confounded with spontaneous recovery, which is greatest in the early months. Also there are plenty of studies showing that later treatment can be just as effective (Wertz *et al.*, 1986; Jones, 1986). The answer is probably that different people need therapy at different points in their recovery. Some may be able to start in the early days following their stroke, while others need time to accommodate to the life changes before language work can begin.

Context

The second question is whether therapy should be administered individually or in groups. Again there is no evidence that one regime is necessarily more effective than the other. Instead there are studies showing that both are useful (Byng, 1988; Bollinger *et al.*, 1993). Of more interest is the type of work which is best tackled by the different regimes. Individual therapy is ideal for working on the specific language impairment, since therapy can be very precisely tailored to the needs of the client. However, group work offers an excellent forum for the development of strategies, since here patients can practise on each other and receive honest feedback from their peers. Groups can also lessen the social isolation of aphasia and help the individual to regain a sense of self-worth (Fawcus, 1992). We might also speculate that groups can encourage the generalization of learnt skills to the wider environment, given that they are much more analogous to 'normal' social interactions than individual therapy.

Frequency and duration of therapy

There is some evidence that intensive therapy is desirable. Brindley *et al.* (1989) compared the outcomes of 'conventional' therapy (1 to 2 hours per week) with those of a 3-month intensive course consisting of 25 hours per week. The results strongly favoured the intensive regime and suggested that it may be better to deliver a patient's therapy in short intensive bursts, rather than through an extended weekly course. However, Brindley's subjects may have benefited from the amount of therapy rather than its intensity. This is also indicated by clinical trials, which typically show a positive relationship between treatment length and efficacy (Basso, 1987). It seems that the *quantity* of therapy is the crucial factor. If we are to help our patients, we must offer them enough time to make a difference.

The role of volunteers

A recent survey of aphasia therapists found that almost half made use of volunteers (Mackenzie *et al.*, 1993). Their duties included delivering therapy, running groups, supporting patients, driving and administration. Volunteers can benefit a service in many ways. They can supplement the therapy offered by the qualified clinician, they support clients socially and can release the therapist from time consuming clinical tasks, such as preparing therapy materials. In some clinics, recovering clients are encouraged to take on a volunteering role, which offers a useful extension to their rehabilitation and provides invaluable encouragement to other clients. Unforeseen gains can also follow. For example, volunteers may mobilize their local pub in support of the clinic and, by talking about their work, help to raise awareness of aphasia in the community.

Despite the benefits, there are anxieties about the use of volunteers. One concern is that volunteers are not given adequate training and supervision. Indeed, the Mackenzie survey found that 21% of the clinicians who used volunteers offered no training. There is also the worry that volunteer administered therapy may be replacing, rather than supplementing, what is provided by the qualified clinician. Again the Mackenzie study found that while most therapists were directing the therapy offered by volunteers, 20% were not.

Used appropriately, volunteers can greatly enhance the quality of the service given to people with dysphasia. However, we must clearly distinguish between the role of the volunteer and the work of the trained clinician. If we fail to do this, cost conscious purchasers may be tempted to replace qualified staff with the cheaper volunteer schemes.

Treatment of articulatory dyspraxia

Not all communication problems after stroke are caused by dysphasia. In some cases there is an articulatory dyspraxia, which disrupts the planned execution of speech. Although dysphasia and dyspraxia are very different, they often co-occur. In these cases the clinician has to decide which disorder to treat. If the aphasia is severe, this will probably be the main focus of therapy, since, without language, speech skills are irrelevant. When aphasia is less severe, the clinician may judge that the disorders are contributing equally to the communication impairment. In this case both aphasia and dyspraxia therapy may be offered.

As in aphasia therapy, treatment for dyspraxia aims directly to lessen the impairment and to compensate for it. When the direct approach is chosen, the primary aim is to improve articulation. Like all therapy, dyspraxia programmes are very hierarchical. For example (in severe cases), the first stage may be to initiate voice, then vowel sounds and finally consonants and consonant clusters. Within these groups, sounds are also graded. Thus among the consonants, nasals, such as 'm' and 'n', are usually easiest and fricatives, such as 's' and 'f' most difficult (Mackenzie, 1982). Of course, hierarchies are varied to take account of individual preferences. Programmes can also be tailored to the client by using personally significant targets, like family names, to introduce new sounds.

Clinicians employ a range of techniques to introduce speech sounds, such as modelling, repetition and explaining how sounds are formed. In some cases it is necessary to help the person form sounds by directly manipulating the articulators. For example, the clinician may guide the patient's tongue tip to the alveolar ridge in order to facilitate a 't' sound. Another cueing technique is known as PROMPT (Prompts for Restructuring Oral Muscular Phonetic Targets, reported in Duffy, 1995). This uses highly structured finger placements on the person's face or neck to stimulate production. For example, cues for the sound 'm' would consist of a finger on the lips to indicate bilabial placement and a thumb on the side of the nose to signal nasality.

Once sounds are established, they usually require considerable practice, or drilling, before they become stabilised. This practice is again hierarchical: for example, Rosenbek *et al.* (1973) suggest an eight step hierarchy, which progresses from direct imitation of the therapist through to the production of words in response to questions or within role plays.

Stress drills can be useful for practising speech sounds (Wertz *et al.*, 1984). Here the therapist and patient indulge in curious dialogues which focus on the target words and sounds. Below is an example of a stress drill for 'kl' clusters:

Therapist: 'Is Nixon the President?'
Patient: 'No *Clinton*.'
Therapist: 'Is Reagan the President?'
Patient: 'No, *Clinton*.'

A number of 'visual aids' can assist dyspraxia therapy, such as pictures of mouth shapes or even vocal tract diagrams, which illustrate the production of sounds. Cued articulation has also been used (Passy, 1990). This is a system of hand signals which accompany speech and provide visible reminders of where and how the sounds are produced. Signs can be made by the therapist, or by the client as a form of a self-cue, although this will be difficult if limb dyspraxia is present. Facilitating gestures may be less explicit. For example, Wertz *et al.* (1984) advocate the use of simple, repetitive movements, such as table tapping, to accompany speech. Explaining why such gestures work is difficult, although they may help the person to slow down and attend to stress and rhythm.

Some therapies exploit the residual skills of dyspraxic people. Occasionally people with dyspraxia can sing the words of songs, although they cannot say them. Melodic Intonation Therapy, which was developed for people with aphasia, aims to capitalize on this skill by encouraging a heavily intoned form of speech (Sparks *et al.*, 1974). Duffy (1995) suggests that this approach may be helpful for some dyspraxic speakers, particularly those who cannot benefit from other techniques.

Other techniques make use of preserved automatic utterances. In one such approach, these stereotyped utterances are carefully modified into new words, thus expanding the speech range of the individual. For example, if the person can only say 'two', this might be shaped into the words 'tie' or 'toe'. A slightly different approach aims to give the person greater voluntary control over these utterances, and hence make them more useful. This may have two benefits: firstly, making planned use of these utterances may generally facilitate propositional speech; secondly, it encourages subjects to make creative use of whatever skills are available. For example, one of our group members used his only utterance, 'boom', to imitate the chimes at the start of a particular news programme, thus conveying what he had watched on TV. Miller (1986) suggests that longer stereotyped utterances can be used as 'carrier phrases or lead-ins' for new sounds and words.

The above techniques all aim directly to improve the articulatory skills of the individual. In contrast, compensatory dyspraxia therapies aim to facilitate communication despite the speech problem. One means of doing this is to encourage alternatives to speech. Here, writing is an obvious choice. However, when aphasia is present, clinicians may have to rely on non-linguistic options, such as gesture. There have been several reports of successful signing therapy with dyspraxic clients. For example, Code and Gaunt (1986) equipped their severely dyspraxic patient with a useful vocabulary of Makaton signs and Skelly *et al.* (1974) facilitated speech through Amer-Ind. Where the dyspraxia is mild, compensatory therapy promotes strategies which reduce articulatory effort. For example, patients may be encouraged to replace phonologically complex words with easier alternatives, or use a telegrammatic style of speaking. Depending on language and motor abilities, people with dyspraxia may be able to supplement speech with computers and other communication aids.

Therapy for dysarthria

Dysarthria differs from dyspraxia in that the speech muscles are paralysed or weak. As with dyspraxia, dysarthria therapy aims to improve speech production and/or compensate for the problem. However, the techniques used are very different. In particular, dysarthria therapy typically places more emphasis on voice and resonance, as these are frequently compromised by the weakened muscles. Another difference is in the use of nonspeech exercises. These are rarely appropriate in dyspraxia, where muscle function is normal. However, they may feature in dysarthria therapy. For example, in spastic dysarthria stretching exercises of the articulators might be attempted to reduce rigidity (Duffy, 1995).

Direct work on speech production will take different forms, depending on the precise nature of the dysarthria. However, a common aim is often to reduce speech rate, as this allows more time for the completion and co-ordination of speech movements. Slowed speech may be promoted through simple aids, such as a pacing board. Yorkston *et al.* (1988) advocates the use of an alphabet board, on which the client points to the first letter of each spoken word. This not only slows speech but also provides the listener with a helpful cue to aid interpretation.

In addition to altering their speech rate, clients may be encouraged to exaggerate, or over-articulate, certain sounds in order to make them clearer. Some people may have to develop new ways of pronouncing sounds, in order to bypass the effects of paralysis. For example, a client who cannot achieve lip closure may learn to produce the bilabial sounds by forming a seal between the tongue and the top lip.

Prosthetic devices can be helpful to some dysarthric speakers. For example, many people with dysarthria cannot achieve velopharyngeal closure, resulting in excessive nasal air flow during speech. In some cases, this can be helped with a palatal lift (designed in collaboration with a prosthodontist), which assists elevation of the soft palate. Voice amplifiers can also be useful in prosthetic therapy, although these are only suitable where articulation has been relatively spared and difficulties are confined to low volume.

Not all dysarthria therapy aims to improve intelligibility. An alternative, or complementary approach aims to develop strategies for coping with the problem. Some strategies may be adopted by the speaker. For example, they may be encouraged to signal the topic before they attempt communication, or provide more redundancy in their speech. Other strategies are adopted by the listener. These might include repeating back what has just been said, thus ensuring comprehension and providing opportunities for repair. An important aspect of strategic therapy is the modification of the physical environment, so that barriers to communication are removed. Typical modifications include the elimination of background noise and adjustments to lighting and seating arrangements.

Dysarthric clients are often good candidates for communication aids, especially when there are no additional cognitive impairments. Keyboard communicators, speech synthesizers and word processors are among the devices used with this group. Where movement is impaired, adapted software, which enables access through a simplified keyboard or mouse, can be particularly useful. Of course high tech solutions are not always best, are expensive, often cumbersome and may saddle the client with an unacceptable synthesized voice. If the client can still use his hands, the old fashioned pencil and paper are hard to beat.

Acknowledgements

This chapter was prepared while the author was supported by MRC Grant Number G 9231810N

References

Basso, A. (1987) Approaches to neuropsychological rehabilitation; language disorders. In *Neuropsychological Rehabilitation* (M. Meier, A. Benton & L. Diller (eds). Churchill Livingstone, London.

Behrmann, M. (1989) The rites of righting writing: homophone remediation in acquired dysgraphia. *Cognitive Neuropsychology* **3**, 365–84.

Behrmann, M. & Lieberthal, T. (1989) Category specific treatment of a lexical-semantic deficit: a single case study of global aphasia. *British Journal of Disorders of Communication* **24**, 281–99.

Bollinger, R., Musson, N. & Holland, A. (1993) A study of group communication intervention with chronically aphasic persons. *Aphasiology* **7**, 301–13.

Borenstein, P. (1993) *Depression and Aphasia*, paper given as the Mary Law Lecture. Action for Dysphasic Adults, London.

Brindley, P., Copeland, M., Demain, C. & Martyn, P. (1989) A comparison of speech of ten chronic Broca's aphasics following intensive and non-intensive periods of therapy. *Aphasiology* **3**, 695–707.

Byng, S. (1988) Sentence processing deficits: theory and therapy. *Cognitive Neuropsychology* **5**, 629–76.

Byng, S. & Coltheart, M. (1986) Aphasia therapy research: methodological requirements and illustrative results. In *Communication and Handicap: Aspects of Psychological Compensation and Technical Aids* (E. Helmquist and L.B. Nilsson, eds). Lawrence Erlbaum, Hillsdale, NJ.

Byng, S. & Jones, E. (1993) *Interactions in therapy*, paper presentation to the British Aphasiology Society Conference, Warwick.

Code, C. & Gaunt, C. (1986) Treating severe speech and limb apraxia in a case of aphasia. *British Journal of Disorders of Communication* **21**, 11–21.

Cubelli, R. (1995) More on drawing in aphasia therapy. *Aphasiology* **9**, 50–6.

David, R., Enderby, P. & Bainton, D. (1982) Treatment of acquired aphasia: speech therapists and volunteers compared. *Journal of Neurology, Neurosurgery and Psychiatry* **45**, 957–61.

De Partz, M.P. (1986) Re-education of a deep dyslexic patient: rational of the method and results. *Cognitive Neuropsychology* **3**, 149–77.

Duffy, J.R. (1995) *Motor Speech Disorders: Substrates, Differential Diagnosis and Management.* Mosby, St. Louis, Missouri.

Fawcus, M. & Lawson, R. (in press) Case Study. In *The Aphasia Treatment File* (S. Byng and E. Jones, eds).

Fawcus, M. (1992) Group work with the aphasic adult. In *Group Encounters in Speech and Language Therapy*. Far Communications, Leicester.

Howard, D. (1986) Beyond randomised controlled trails: the case for effective case studies of the effects of treatment in aphasia. *British Journal of Disorders of Communication* **21**, 89–102.

Jones, E. (1986) Building the foundations of sentence production in a non-fluent aphasic. *British Journal of Disorders of Communication* **21**, 63–82.

Jones, E. (1989) *A Year in the Life of EVJ and PC*, proceedings of the Summer Conference of the British Aphasiology Society, Cambridge.

Jones, E. & Byng, S. (1988) The practice of aphasia therapy: an opinion. *Bulletin of the College of Speech Therapists* No. 449, 2–4.

Kagan, A. & Gailey, G. (1993) Functional is not enough: training conversation partners for aphasic adults. In *Aphasia Treatment: World Perspectives* (A.L. Holland and M.M. Forbes, eds). Chapman and Hall, London.

Kinsella, G. & Duffy, F. (1978) The spouse of the aphasic patient. In *The Management of Aphasia* (Y. Lubrun and R. Hoops, eds). Swets and Zeitlinger, Amsterdam.

Lesser, R. & Algar, L. (1995) Towards combining the cognitive neuropsychological and the pragmatic in aphasia therapy. *Neuropsychological Rehabilitation* **5**, 67–92.

Lincoln, N., McGuirk, E., Mulley, G., Lendrem, W., Jones, A. & Mitchell, J. (1984) Effectiveness of speech therapy for aphasic stroke patients: a randomised controlled trial. *Lancet* **1**, 1197–1200.

Lyon, J. (1995) Drawing: its value as a communication aid for adults with aphasia. *Aphasiology* **9**, 33–50.

Lyon, J. (1995) Communicative drawing: an augmentative mode of interaction. *Aphasiology* **9**, 84–94.

Mackenzie, C. (1982) Aphasic articulatory defect and aphasic phonological defect. *British Journal of Disorder of Communication* **17**, 27–46.

Mackenzie, C., Le May, M., Lendrem, W., McGuirk, E., Marshall, J. & Rossiter, D. (1993) A survey of aphasia services in the United Kingdom. *European Journal of Disorders of Communication* **28**, 43–63.

Marshall, J. (1989) *RS: Three Specific Treatment Programmes*, proceedings of the Summer Conference of the British Aphasiology Society, Cambridge.

Marshall, J. (1995) The mapping hypothesis and aphasia therapy. *Aphasiology* **9**, 517–39.

Marshall, J., Pound, C., White-Thomson, M. & Pring, T. (1990) The use of the picture/word matching tasks to assist word retrieval in aphasic patients. *Aphasiology* **4**, 167–84.

Marshall, J., Chiat, S. & Pring, T. (1997) An impairment in processing verbs' thematic roles: a therapy study. *Aphasiology* **11**, 855–76.

McIntosh, J. & Dakin, G. (1989) *Restoration of Communication Through Amer-Ind*, proceedings of the Summer Conference of the British Aphasiology Society, Cambridge.

Meikle, M., Wechsler, E., Tupper, A., Benenson, M., Butler, J., Mulhall, D. & Stern, G. (1979) Comparative trial of volunteer and professional treatments of dysphasia after stroke. *BMJ* **2**, 87–9.

Miller, N. (1986) *Dyspraxia and Its Management*. Croom Helm, London.

Mulhull, D. (1978) Dysphasic stroke patients and the influence of their relatives. *British Journal of Disorders of Communication* **13**, 127–34.

Nettleton, J. & Lesser, R. (1991) Application of a cognitive neuropsychological model to therapy for naming difficulties. *Journal of Neurolinguistics* **6**, 139–57.

Nickels, L., Byng, S. & Black, M. (1991) Sentence Processing Deficits: a replication of therapy. *British Journal of Disorders of Communication* **26**, 139–57.

Nickels, L. & Best, W. (1994) Therapy for naming deficits: specifics, surprises and suggestions. *Aphasiology* **10**, 21–47.

Passy, J. (1990) *Cued Articulation; A Handbook of Cues*.

Pring, T. (1986) Evaluating the effects of speech therapy for aphasics: developing the single case methodology. *British Journal of Disorder of Communication* **21**, 103–15.

Pring, T., White-Thomson, M., Pound, C., Marshall, J. & Davis, A. (1990) Picture/word matching tasks and word retrieval: Some follow up data and second thoughts. *Aphasiology* **4**, 479–83.

Rosenbek, J.C. *et al.* (1973) A treatment for apraxia of speech in adults. *Journal of Speech and Hearing Disorders* **38**, 462.

Sands, E., Sarno, M. & Shankweiler, D. (1969) Long-term assessment of language function in aphasia due to stroke. *Archives of Physical Medicine and Rehabilitation* **52**, 73–8.

Scott, C. & Byng, S. (1989) Computer assisted remediation of a homophone comprehension disorder in surface dyslexia. *Aphasiology* **3**, 301–20.

Skelly, M. (1979) *American Indian Gestural Code.* Elsevier, North Holland, New York.

Skelly, M., Sehinsky, L., Smith, R. & Fust, R. (1974) American Indian sign (Amerind) as a facilitator of verbalisation for the oral–verbal apractic. *Journal of Speech and Hearing Disorders* **39**, 445–456.

Sparks, R., Helm, N. & Albert, M. (1974) Aphasia rehabilitation resulting from Melodic Intonation Therapy. *Journal of Speech and Hearing Disorders* **41**, 287–97.

Wertz, R., LaPoint, L. & Rosenbek, J. (1984) Apraxia of Speech in Adults: The Disorder and Its Management. F. Grune and Stratton, Orlando, Fl.

Wertz, R., Weiss, D., Aten, L., Brookshire, R., Carcia-Bunuel, L., Holland, A., Kurtzke, J., Greenbaum, H., Marshall, R., Vogel, D., Carter, J., Barnes, N. & Goodman, R. (1986) Comparison of clinic, home and deferred language treatment for aphasia: a VA Co-operative study. *Archives of Neurology* **43**, 653–58.

Whitehead, S. (1992) Support groups for the relatives or carers of aphasic adults. In *Group Encounters in Speech and Language Therapy* (M. Fawcus, ed.). Far Communication, Leicester.

Yorkston, K.M., Beukelman, D. & Bell, K. (1988) *Clinical Management of Dysarthric Speakers.* College-Hill Press, San Diego, Ca.

Chapter 9

Rehabilitation of Cognitive and Emotional Problems Following Stroke

Simon B.N. Thompson

Several definitions of stroke have been used in the past (Aho *et al.*, 1980; Isaacs, 1983). It is important to realize the consequences of these definitions and to understand two central features: that is, the sudden rapid onset (which has a devastating effect on the stroke victim) and the site of disturbance – the brain (the central control system for the whole body).

The brain is the most complex organ of the body, and as such, damage to different areas will cause varying functional deficits. Brain cells are usually considered irreplaceable compared to other tissue areas that can reproduce as necessary. However, the possibilities of brain plasticity (the ability of brain cells to take over the function of the damaged areas) have been investigated (Raisman & Field, 1973; Wall, 1980; Bach-y-Rita, 1981).

Prognosis

In any rehabilitation process, it is important to discern which aspects of a patient's medical history may have contributed to his/her disability. In order to understand the extent of the disability, it is helpful to acquire an understanding of the anatomical sites that affect function. Knowledge of such cerebral function and circulation greatly assists both therapists and medical staff in interpreting the symptomatology in order to determine the extent of the stroke and the areas involved (Thompson & Morgan, 1995). For example, the functions normally associated with the frontal lobe are intellect, emotions, behaviour, language, personality, control centres for higher autonomic functions, abstract thinking and motor movement (Goetter, 1986). The parietal lobe is responsible for reception, perception, and interpretation of sensory information including touch, pain, temperature, pressure, size, shape and awareness of space (Rose & Capildeo, 1981; Sharpless, 1982). Alterations in blood flow through the internal carotid, middle cerebral, and anterior cerebral arteries produce dysfunction of the frontal and parietal lobes.

Generally, the more severe the impairment or disability is initially, the more severe will be the disability at six months. Many studies have identified individual impairments which are associated with more severe disabilities at six months, including hemianopia, severe sensory loss, complete motor loss, loss of trunk balance, loss of consciousness, presence of neglect, and presence of confusion (Wade, 1993). Additionally, urinary incontinence after a stroke is a good indicator of a poor outcome (Barer, 1989), and various attempts have been made at quantifying outcome in order to predict prognosis according to probability and therapy (Allen, 1984; Thompson, 1987; Thompson & Coleman, 1987, 1988).

Cognition

Cognition is a general term often used to describe the thinking and mental processes of the brain. Depending on the specific sites of brain damage, those areas of the brain responsible for cognitive aspects of brain functioning (as compared with physical and sensory functions) will be affected to varying degrees. Confusion following a stroke is especially common (Isaacs, 1983), and with older patients, this is even more common and can be alarming for the individual affected. It can also be difficult to resolve. Patients who are unaware of time- or space-orientation may become distressed if they cannot understand where they are, or their purpose in that particular place. This may lead to wandering, difficulty in finding their way home, or a lack of recognition of visitors (even relatives) or staff. Therefore, it becomes especially important for carers to allow patients to become gently orientated to their often new and strange environment, especially if it is an unfamiliar hospital ward.

Intelligence

Intelligence is a term that has been variously defined. However, it is generally regarded as the way an individual functions in terms of his/her mental processes or cognitions. Hence, more usefully, clinicians refer to a person's 'intellectual functioning' (Thompson & Morgan, 1995) and try to find out which aspects or functions are better than others. In the case of the stroke patient, this may mean testing the patient's concentration on a set of specific tasks or asking the patient to add together a series of numerical values, etc.

The clinician aims to gather information on all aspects of the patient's functioning in order to establish which abilities may have been affected and therefore, which areas of the brain have sustained impairment. Sometimes it is by process of elimination of different possible test outcomes, and sometimes it is by gaining an overall picture of the patient's presentation (which includes a clinical interview with the patient and relatives or carers) that these conclusions can be made.

Typically, several neuropsychological tests are administered to cover abilities such as immediate and delayed memory, recognition and recall, ability to shift set in problem-solving tasks, verbal fluency and arithmetic-type tasks.

Examples of such tests include the Wechsler Memory Scale (Wechsler, 1987) which aims to assess a number of aspects of a person's memory (e.g. memory for spoken instructions; pattern recognition; memory for digits; memory for diagrams and spatial orientation). Other tests of a neuropsychological assessment battery may include the Recognition Memory Test (Warrington, 1984) which tests recognition of words and people's faces; or tests of memory for everyday objects (Lezak, 1983). Verbal fluency tests include the FAS test (Benton *et al.*, 1983) or the Graded Naming Test (McKenna & Warrington, 1983) which tap vocabulary knowledge but are generally considered to be dependent on a person's post-education and culture. The Wechsler Adult Intelligence Scale (WAIS) and WAIS-R (Revised edition) (Wechsler, 1955, 1981) assess a range of abilities including verbal and performance skills such as visuospatial ability and problem solving. Ability to shift cognitive sets can be assessed by the Wisconsin Card Sorting Test (Heaton *et al.*, 1993) which can highlight problems with cognitive processes often associated with the frontal lobe regions of the brain.

In addition, perceptual testing (e.g. visual neglect tests such as star cancelling or letter identification and cancelling) can also reveal deficits such as hemianopia where half of the visual field is apparently lost in terms of processing. The patient may leave half a plate of food or only attempt to dress the unaffected half of the body. This would be highlighted in specific perceptual testing. Dexterity tests can also help to pin-point deficits in fine motor functioning and overestimation in pointing.

Concentration

Stroke patients often have poor concentration, usually immediately after the stroke. This can impede the rehabilitation process. Therefore, there is a need to breakdown tasks into small stages of achievement as well as grade them in time. Dressing and undressing routines, for example, should be made simpler by setting tasks for the patient to fully complete before moving on to the next task in order to complete the routine as a whole.

Where patients are referred having suffered a stroke many years previously, established routines of one-handed independence may be apparent. In these cases, complete revision of techniques will be unnecessary and difficult to attain, as the patient is unlikely to be willing or unable to 'unlearn' old, familiar techniques. This is where both the clinical neuropsychologist and occupational therapist can work together in a team approach, addressing activities of daily living but specifically seeking to establish sequences of behaviour, whether learned or re-learned, using aide-memoires and reinforcers. Poor concentration also carries with it associated problems such as confusion, frustration and more obvious 'exhibitions' of difficulties such as swearing, shouting and attempts to abscond from a hospital ward or rehabilitation unit. These problems may stem from a lack of understanding of the current situation following poor communication or poor attention to tasks rather than from stubbornness or frustration.

Depression and anxiety

Depression is perhaps an understandable consequence of the sometimes devastating deficits resulting from a stroke. Various methods of assessing depression have been used including the Hospital Anxiety and Depression Scale (Zigmond & Snaith, 1983) and the Beck Depression Inventory (Beck, 1978). However, both depression and anxiety should be assessed over different sessions, in order to observe the patient at different times and carrying out different tasks. The clinical interview, however, is of paramount importance and should always accompany any paper-and-pencil type assessment of the patient's mental status.

Various methods may be used to alleviate depression and anxiety. Apart from drug applications, which may be useful especially in 'taking the edge' off anxiety symptoms, cognitive therapy is by far the most successful. (The reader is referred to Blackburn & Davidson, 1990, for a comprehensive account of cognitive therapy.) Other interventions include supportive counselling and monitoring of behavioural symptoms, which are usually helpful and often accompany cognitive therapy. Very often stroke patients become confused and disorientated. It is worthwhile assessing and reassuring patients whilst attempting to distinguish between the symptoms of depression versus a confusional state, since depression often affects concentration, sometimes followed by disorientation and confusion.

Memory loss

In addition to confusional states following a stroke, loss of memory is also very common. It can be very frustrating to the stroke patient and can be dangerous in the home setting if it is not recognized and taken into account; for example, leaving cookers on or unattended. Memory loss also slows down the rehabilitation process as patients cannot remember the sequence of tasks. Similarly, re-learning can be much more difficult if those parts of the brain responsible for short-term memory have been affected.

Frequent orientation to time and place again become essential for the stroke patient whose short-term memory has been affected. Very often associated deficits are apparent with a patient's poor memory. Common problems include: forgetting lists of words (for example, a shopping list); forgetting names of objects (even for objects frequently used); forgetting past memories, such as those from childhood; forgetting people's names (or names and faces);

forgetting personal details (such as their age or even their name); forgetting what the day or time is or what to do next; forgetting something they have just read; and forgetting words that need to be remembered. All of these can be very disturbing to those who are closest to patients who have these sorts of problems. The results of research (Thompson, 1995; 1996) have found the following steps useful for sufferers of a poor memory, particularly the elderly and those who have had a stroke. They may help to alleviate or even reduce some of the burdens of having problems such as dysphasia and impaired memory, for example, and have been incorporated into a booklet which references a number of useful sources (McKenzie, Thompson & Weeks, 1991).

The following boxes detail strategies that can be used in a variety of situations to help a stroke patient cope with the effects of memory loss.

- To remember a list of words, each word should be illustrated with a familiar household object: for example, the word 'carrot' is pictured watching television; 'sausages' are pictured taking a bath.
- When the words and pictures are well learned, go through the house in your mind picturing each piece of furniture and try to remember the word related to it.

Fig. 9.1 Remembering a list of words.

- Get someone to tell you the word for an object: for example, a cup *when* you use it for drinking.
- In this way, every time you use the cup, you will know what it is called and the words for what you do with it.
- You can also do this exercise by using pictures of objects and repeating the names over and over again.
- The more times you do this, the better.

Fig. 9.2 Remembering names of objects.

- Often things are linked with the past, such as smells or colours during childhood, which can bring back memories when they are experienced again.
- Listening to a record or reading out a poem remembered from childhood may stimulate someone' memory.

Fig. 9.3 Using memories.

- Write the first letter of the name of a person you want to remember on a piece of card.
- When you want to recall the name, look at the card and try to remember the name that begins with that first letter.

Fig. 9.4 Remembering people's names.

- Something that stands out or is unusual about a person's name should be pictured as a mental image. It might be that the person's name stands for a trade, like 'Cooper', which originally meant a 'barrel-maker'.
- Alternatively, there might be something about the person that produces a picture in your mind when you hear the name: this picture should be learned so that it can be used to remember the person's name.

Fig. 9.5   Remembering people's names and faces.

- One way to remember a list of details about a person (such as their name, how old they are or where they live) is to make up a song or a lyric so that you can say it to yourself everytime you want to remember the information.
- It is important to rehearse the lyric several times until you can remember it on a number of occasions without as much help from others.

Fig. 9.6   Forgetting personal details.

- Choose a time in the day when you regularly look at a calendar or a clock, for example, as soon as you get up in the morning.
- Write the date on a piece of card in large sized print and stick it on the wall in the kitchen or somewhere you use regularly. This will remind you of the date.
- It is helpful if someone else can ask you what time it is, or ask what day it is, so that you can rehearse these facts several times during the day. This helps improve 'orientation' for the date and the time of day.

Fig. 9.7   Remembering the date and time of day.

- 'Self-statements' or sentences said to yourself are invented for a particular problem. For example, if you have difficulty remembering what to buy next, make a list of the items before you go shopping and choose a shop (for example, the supermarker) that you will go into if you forget what to do next.
- Then practice saying, 'I'll go into the supermarket whenever I forget the things I came for, and then I'll look at my shopping list.'

Fig. 9.8   Remembering what to do next.

Sometimes, you may forget an article you have just read in the newspaper, or you may forget the gist or meaning of what you have read in a book. The answer to this problem may be the 'PQRST' method:

- P is for preview: read the article fairly quickly so that you know roughly what it is about.
- Q is for question: ask yourself some questions about the article.
- R is for read: read the article again slowly and try to answer the questions as you do this.
- S is for state: say to yourself (or out loud) what the articleis about
- T is for test: now, answer those questions again.
- It will gradually get easier to remember articles if the 'PQRST' method is practiced several times.

Fig. 9.9   Remembering what you have just read.

- Put the words you want to remember in an unusual sentence. Practice saying the sentence.
- When you want to remember the words, try and remember to say the unusual sentence.
- Alternatively, if you want to remember pairs of words (for example, 'up and down') then picture them in your mind: a person going up and down a staircase, on a see-saw, or an image that is clear for you to remember.
- When you want to remember the words, try to remember the picture of them.

Fig. 9.10 Remembering words.

- Keep a clock with a large clear dial on view.
- Keep a calendar handy that can be changed for the day, month, and year.
- Label the doors of all the rooms in your home: the bedroom, bathroom, kitchen, living room, and closets.
- Keep photographs of familiar people, such as your family, on view.
- Leave everyday possessions nearby in handy places. Always keep them in the same location.
- Keep furniture in the same place.
- Make a list of things to do so that you or your helpers can tick them off as they are done.
- Set out things to do in the order in which they have to be done.
- Organize the things you need to use: for example, leave out only one day's medication supply. Label the medications by the times of the day that you need to take them.
- When going out, leave the address of the place you are going to on a piece of paper so that friends or helpers know where you have gone.
- Stick to a routine as far as possible.
- Use a noticeboard to display information you want to remember.

Fig. 9.11 Useful tips to help with a poor memory.

Recognition

Recognizing familiar faces (for example, next of kin or close relatives) is sometimes affected following a stroke (Thompson & Morgan, 1995). This is distressing both to the individual affected and to the relatives of the stroke patient. Sometimes names of previously familiar people are forgotten. This may be due to the failure to recognize a person's face; and sometimes it is an intermittent failure to recognize both names and faces and is very often tied in with the confusion. Such forms of recognition failures are well understood (Thompson & Morgan, 1995), and there are a number of neuropsychological assessments available to test for these (e.g. the Recognition Memory Test – Warrington, 1984).

Some patients may experience difficulty in naming familiar objects following a stroke. Depending on the site of brain damage patients may also have problems expressing or understanding language.

Emotion

Emotional lability, fear and denial of disability are examples of common psychological problems in the early stages of recovery from a stroke and are often coupled with confusion (Thompson & Morgan, 1995). Inappropriate laughter or crying can be very disconcerting to other ward patients and relatives. These need to be treated with patience and tolerance, as the patient will usually be unaware of his/her plight. Fear of the future, which often leads to denial of any problem, can also occur and again requires reassurance, explanation and a sympathetic approach.

More severe psychological effects such as anxiety, agitation, or clinical depression, requires more specific intervention. A patient who is severely depressed will lack motivation to perform even the simplest of tasks, such as maintaining posture, attempting communication, etc. (Ebrahim, 1985; Collin *et al.*, 1987). Similarly, a patient who is overanxious or extremely agitated will not be able to settle to the routine and demands of the rehabilitation programme. In these cases, psychiatric assessment and treatment enables the continuation of the rehabilitation process.

As Hermann and Wallesch (1993) have stated, consideration of depressive changes following stroke is becoming more important both for research and for rehabilitation. The success of rehabilitation may depend on early diagnosis and adequate therapy, and these facts have been demonstrated on a number of occasions (Robinson *et al.*, 1984, 1986; Parikh, 1988). Both primary and secondary depression have a negative effect on motivation and progress in the first four to six months post-stroke when rehabilitation treatment is most promising. Depression may account for impaired compliance and lack of progress, which in turn may contribute to increased depression (Hermann & Wallesch, 1993). These factors tend to confound results of testing patients with strokes, especially when attendance on a specific assessment task is important to discern a particular deficit. The emotional consequences, therefore, have considerable impact on the patient; and reactions such as grief-responses and depression should be borne in mind when making both the initial assessment of the stroke patient, as well as during rehabilitation. The reader is referred to the wealth of literature on emotional reactions following stroke (Schwabb, 1972; Folstein *et al.*, 1977; Charatan & Fiosk, 1978).

Psychosocial effects

Language disorders are very common and often follow a stroke. They are not always permanent, but often there is a residual deficit even after a period of speech therapy. These deficits cause considerable distress to the stroke patient and family and contribute to the patient's loss of self-esteem or self-worth. As well as making it difficult for family members to communicate or understand the patient, language disorders sometimes create a psychological 'distance' between close relatives and patients. By building up a better understanding of these problems for relatives (as well as for the patient) through counselling – whether psycho-educational or through more directive approaches such as psychodynamic therapy – the whole family becomes better equipped psychologically to support the patient.

Psychosocial effects following stroke can follow sexual dysfunction. Changes in perception can also lead to confusion and misinterpretation of environmental stimuli, which in turn develop into a psychosocial problem for the patient. To function again as a member of the family or as part of the peer group, the patient has to overcome an immediate feeling of 'denial' and address the specific issues concerning him/herself. Social acceptability can be difficult to achieve in a society that still stigmatizes disability to a certain extent. Therefore, the long-term psychological consequences of a stroke need to be addressed. These are often confronted through counselling or consultation with a clinical neuropsychologist.

Therapeutic approaches

The treatment of stroke patients has become a subject of much controversy in recent years. Developments in our knowledge of stroke have led to changing attitudes to this area of medicine. The conventional unilateral approach left many patients completely one-sided and one-handed but also relatively, if not completely, dependent (Thompson & Morgan, 1995). A key proponent of the holistic approach to the treatment of stroke was Bobath (1985). Research into neurophysiological techniques has revealed that conventional approaches are not necessarily the best for the patient. However, until enough therapists become familiar with these new techniques, occupational therapy education in particular will remain biased towards more conventional treatment methods.

Psychological support

As well as assessing clinically the range of abilities remaining with the affected stroke patient, there is considerable support available for the psychological welfare of the patient, in the form of counselling or therapy/advice from the rehabilitation team. Apart from assistance and advice concerning memory and concentration, there is the issue of bereavement and the change in lifestyle following the initial trauma of suffering a stroke. These issues are often addressed by a clinical neuropsychologist attached to a stroke unit or as part of a general hospital department.

Denial is common among stroke patients and surrounds issues of inability to perform previously easy or well-learned tasks. There can be a sense of bereavement for those lost skills, and there can be disproportionation (i.e. a distortion of true perspective) for the extent of loss. A number of psychological approaches can be offered for such patients by the clinical psychologist and include: cognitive therapy; cognitive-behavioural therapy; advice for specific difficulties such as memory loss and counselling. Cognitive therapy is fundamentally a 'talking therapy' and aims to establish what perceptions the patient has and to expose their irrational beliefs. Tackling each belief in turn, this approach attempts to seek evidence for and against those beliefs held by the patient and for them to progress by overcoming any fears or refuting unreal values. Cognitive-behavioural therapy incorporates behavioural elements in an approach by using techniques to modify or change the patient's behaviour. This may be carried out through keeping a diary of an individual's behaviour or by shaping the incorrect behaviour through reinforcement (Blackburn & Davidson, 1990).

Counselling

Counselling is a term often used to describe a number of different approaches. This is most often meant to imply work of a supportive nature for patients and can address an individual's fears or problems as a result of a stroke. By discussing and reflecting on values held, the individual is often guided by the therapist into solving problems by providing their own solutions through the direction of the therapist. However, counselling can be interpreted in many different ways and can also imply a less-directive, nonstructured route to problem solving or simply to provide a 'listening ear' for the patient.

A number of problems may be encountered during a counselling session. Sometimes the patient feels inhibited perhaps because of the personal nature of his/her disclosures or perhaps if there is not a good rapport between patient and therapist. It is important for the therapist to establish trust in the therapeutic relationship early on so that the patient feels comfortable and can be moved on in the therapy session. Clinical psychologists spend varying amounts of time during their training learning different approaches to interviewing patients and matching the most appropriate therapeutic intervention to each patient and situation. Some psychologists regard much of their work as imparting advice and information other than counselling patients, but others in the profession see counselling as a key component of therapy.

Communicating well in counselling sessions is paramount, and it is often necessary to find the level at which the patient communicates and understands; for example, jargonistic or patronizing language is to be avoided and listening and reflecting back the patient's feelings and views is a more useful practice in order to establish acceptable communication by both patient and therapist. Where possible and where appropriate, humour can be a useful relief to a therapy session, but likewise 'staying' with a patient's emotion (especially if the patient weeps) is also useful in order to explore further how the patient is feeling about a particular problem at that time. Sometimes these emotions provide an ideal opportunity to explore sensitive issues such as the patient's fears and to convey empathy with the patient or to establish an understanding of the patient's condition.

Research continues into the different therapeutic approaches involved in the rehabilitation process for the stroke patient, and several interesting papers have addressed common issues such as the problems with activities of daily living (ADL), outcome of therapeutic approaches, and survival rates of stroke victims

(Thompson & Coleman, 1987; Langton-Hewer, 1990; Shah *et al.*, 1990; Thorngren *et al.*, 1990). With ever advancing technology both in industry and in medicine, there is renewed hope for recovery of cerebral functions following stroke.

References

Aho, K., Harmsen, P., Hatano, S., Marquarsden, J., Smirnov, V.E. *et al.* (1980) Cerebrovascular disease in the community: results of a collaborative study. *Bulletin of the World Health Organization* **58**, 113–30.

Allen, C.M.C. (1984) Predicting the outcome of acute stroke: a prognostic score. *Journal of Neurology, Neurosurgery and Psychiatry* **47**, 475–80.

Bach-y-Rita, P. (1981) Brain plasticity as a basis for the development of rehabilitation procedures for hemiplegia. *Scandinavian Journal of Rehabilitation Medicine* **13**, 73–83.

Barer, E.H. (1989) Continence after stroke – useful predictor or goal of therapy? *Age and Ageing* **18**, 183–91.

Beck, A.T. (1978) *Beck Depression Inventory*. Harcourt Brace Jovanovich, San Antonio.

Benton, A.L., Hamsher, K. de S., Varney, N.R. & Spreen, O. (1983) *Contributions to Neuropsychological Assessment*. Oxford University Press, New York.

Blackburn, I.M. & Davidson, K. (1990) *Cognitive Therapy for Depression and Anxiety: A Practitioner's Guide*. Blackwell, Oxford.

Bobath, B. (1985) *Adult Hemiplegia: Evaluation and Treatment*. Heinemann, London.

Charatan, F.B. & Fiosk, A. (1978) Mental and emotional results of stroke. *New York State Journal of Medicine* **78**, 1403–5.

Collin, S.T., Tinson, D. & Lincoln, N.B. (1987) Depression and stroke. *Disability and Rehabilitation* **1**, 27–32.

Ebrahim, S. (1985) Depression after stroke: A common cause of rehabilitation failure. *Geriatric Medicine* **15**(7), 5–6.

Folstein, M.F., Maiberger, R. & McHugh, P.R. (1977) Mood disorder as a specific complication of stroke. *Journal of Neurology, Neurosurgery and Psychiatry* **40**, 1018–20.

Goetter, W. (1986) Nursing diagnoses and interventions with the acute stroke patient. *Nursing Clinics of North America* **21**(2), 309–19.

Heaton, R.K., Chelune, G.J., Talley, J.L., Kay, G.G. & Curtiss, G. (1993) *Wisconsin Card Sorting Manual Revised and Expanded*. Psychological Assessment Resources, Florida.

Hermann, M. & Wallesch, C.-W. (1993) Depressive changes in stroke patients. *Disability and Rehabilitation* **15**(2), 55–66.

Isaacs, B. (1983) *Understanding Stroke Illness*. Chest, Heart and Stroke Association, London.

Langton-Hewer, R. (1990) Rehabilitation after stroke. *Quarterly Journal of Medicine (New Series)* **76**, 659–74.

Lezak, M.D. (1983) *Neuropsychological Assessment*, 2nd edn, pp. 330–1. Oxford University Press, New York.

McKenna, P. & Warrington, E.K. (1983) *Graded Naming Test*. NFER-Nelson, Windsor.

McKenzie, K., Thompson, S.B.N. & Weeks, D.J. (1991) *Your Memory Manual: A Self-Help Guide to Help Overcome Everyday Memory Difficulties*. Lothian Health Board, Edinburgh.

Parikh, R.M., Lipsey, J.R., Robinson, R.G. & Price, T.R. (1998) A two-year longitudinal study of post-stroke mood disorders: prognostic factors related to one and two year outcome. *International Journal of Psychiatry in Medicine* **18**, 45–56.

Raisman, G. & Field, P.M. (1973) A quantitative investigation of the development of collateral renervation of the septal nuclei. *Brain Research* **50**, 241–64.

Robinson, R.G., Lipsey, J.R., Rao, K. & Price, T.R. (1986) Two year longitudinal study of post-stroke mood disorders: comparison of acute-onset with delayed-onset depression. *American Journal of Psychiatry* **143**, 1238–44.

Robinson, R.G., Starr, L.B., Lipsey, J.R., Rao, K. & Price, T.R. (1984) A two-year longitudinal study of post-stroke mood disorders: dynamic changes in associated variables over the first six months of follow-up. *Stroke* **15**, 510–17.

Ross, F. & Capildeo, R. (1981) *Stroke, the Facts.* Oxford University Press, New York.

Schwabb, J.J. (1972) Emotional considerations in cancer and stroke. *New York State Journal of Medicine* **72**, 2877–80.

Shah, S., Venclay, F. & Cooper, B. (1990) Efficiency, effectiveness, and duration of stroke rehabilitation. *Stroke* **21**, 241–6.

Sharpless, J.W. (1982) *Mossman's Problem-Oriented Approach to Stroke Rehabilitation,* 2nd edn. Charles C. Thomas, Springfield, Illinois.

Thompson, S.B.N. (1995) Storage problems. *Therapy Weekly* **21**(40), 7.

Thompson, S.B.N. (1996) Practical ways of improving memory storage and retrieval problems in patients with head injuries. *British Journal of Occupational Therapy* **59**(9), 418–22.

Thompson, S.B.N. (1987) A microcomputer-based assessment battery, data file handling and data retrieval system for the forward planning of treatment for adult stroke patients. *Journal of Microcomputer Applications* **10**(2), 127–35.

Thompson, S.B.N. & Coleman, M.J. (1987) Stroke recovery model. *Therapy Weekly* **14**(9), 7.

Thompson, S.B.N. & Coleman, M.J. (1988) Occupational therapists' prognoses of their patients: findings of a British survey of stroke. *International Journal of Rehabilitation Research* **11**(3), 275–9.

Thompson, S.B.N. & Morgan, M. (1995) *Occupational Therapy for Stroke Rehabilitation.* Chapman and Hall, London.

Thorngren, M., Westling, B. & Norrving, B. (1990) Outcome after stroke in patients discharged to independent living. *Stroke* **21**, 236–40.

Wade, D. (1993) Stroke. In *Neurological Rehabilitation* (R. Greenwood *et al.*, eds), pp. 451–8. Churchill Livingstone, Edinburgh.

Wall, P.D. (1980) Mechanisms of plasticity connection following damage in adult mammalian nervous systems. *Recovery of Function: Theoretical Considerations for Brain Injury Rehabilitation* (P. Bach-y-Rita, ed.), pp. 91–105. University Park Press, Baltimore.

Warrington, E.K. (1984) *Recognition Memory Test.* NFER-Nelson, Windsor.

Wechsler, D. (1955) *Wechsler Adult Intelligence Scale.* The Psychological Corporation, San Antonio.

Wechsler, D. (1981) *Wechsler Adult Intelligence Scale – Revised Manual.* The Psychological Corporation, San Antonio.

Wechsler, D. (1987) *Wechsler Memory Scale – Revised Manual.* Harcourt Brace Jovanovich, San Antonio.

Zigmond, A.S. & Snaith, P. (1983) The Hospital Anxiety and Depression Scale. *Acta Psychiatrika Scandinavika* **67**, 361–70.

Further Reading

Collin, M.E. (1975) Neurophysiological techniques in the treatment of adult neurologically impaired patients. *British Journal of Occupational Therapy* **8**, 166–7.

Korner-Bitensky, N., Mayo, N.E. & Kaizer, F. (1990) Changes in response time of stroke patients and controls during rehabilitation. *American Journal of Physical Medicine and Rehabilitation* **69**, 32–8.

Parikh, R.M., Robinson, R.G., Lipsey, J.R. & Starkstein, S.E. (1990) The impact of post-stroke depression on recovery in activities of daily living over a 2-year follow-up. *Archives of Neurology* **47**, 785–9.

Starkstein, S.E., Cohen, B.S., Federoff, P., Parikh, R.M., Price, T.R. & Robinson, R.G. (1990) Relationship between anxiety disorders and depressive disorders in patients with cerebrovascular injury. *Archives of General Psychiatry* **47**, 246–51.

Stern, R.A. & Bachman, D.L. (1991) Depressive symptoms following stroke. *American Journal of Psychiatry* **148**, 351–6.

Thompson, S.B.N. & Coleman, M.J. (1988) Making the therapist's prognosis of stroke a more scientific process. In *Information Technology and Human Services* (B. Glastonbury, W. La Mendola & S. Toole, eds), pp. 68–75. John Wiley, Chichester.

Wade, D.R., Leigh-Smith, J.E. & Hewer, R.A. (1987) Depressed mood after stroke, a community study of its frequency. *British Journal of Psychiatry* **151**, 200–5.

Chapter 10

Personal Construct Theory in Stroke and Communication Problems

Shelagh Brumfitt

There is still confusion over what constitutes a natural emotional response to the stroke, and how this ties in with the neurological effects on the brain which may cause a change in personality or emotional state (Rollin, 1987; Code, 1993). However, most authors acknowledge that depression and feelings of hopelessness about the future are significant effects which need attention. Anderson (1992) reports the lack of attention to treatment of emotional and social consequences of stroke. Mulley (1985) discusses the psychological effects of stroke by using a model of grief. He attributes depression in the early stages as being part of the grief reaction, but notes that the greatest degree of depression can occur between six months and two years post-onset. Robinson *et al.* (1987) differentiated the evolution of major and minor depression during the first two years after a stroke. Patients with major depression improved significantly between years one and two. In contrast, patients with minor depression did not demonstrate such improvement, and some actually developed major depression by the two-year follow-up. Robinson *et al.* conclude that major depression appears to have a natural course of approximately one year, while minor depression frequently has a longer course.

With this increased awareness of the psychological impact, there have been recent changes of emphasis in the development of services for the person who has suffered stroke. Niemi *et al.* (1988) studied quality of life in forty-six stroke survivors four years after their stroke. Their lives were studies in terms of working conditions, activities at home, family relationships and leisure time activities. It was shown that in spite of a good recovery in terms of discharge from hospital, activities of daily living, and return to work, the quality of life of most patients (83%) had not been restored to the pre-stroke level. Deterioration among the several domains of life ranged from 39% to 80%, the lowest being in the domain of activities at home and the highest in the domain of leisure time activities. This recognition of quality of life issues has facilitated the improved approach to helping people with stroke conditions.

In the past there have been different approaches used to meet this need.

There have been recent moves to conceptualize the effects of stroke within a social model as opposed to the traditional medical model. That is, the environment or social context in which the individual exists is viewed as a critical factor in the way the individual responds to stroke. If the WHO typology of impairment, disability and handicap is used as a model, then impairment level therapy is concerned with the actual damage to the body, the disability level is concerned with assisting the individual with performance of activities and everyday functioning, and the handicap level refers to the psychological and social consequences of living with the impairment and disability. What is useful about this model is that it 'permits' the professional to recognize the emotional and psychological needs of the individual. Giving attention to this area may facilitate improved coping strategies in the individual and empower stroke patients as a social group.

Bury (1982) refers to the onset of chronic illness as constituting a 'biographical disruption' which calls into question both the individual's past experiences and present experiences. This has implications for the self-concept. At no notice the individual is forced to review self within the new context (i.e. being a chronically ill person). Charmaz (1995) discusses the threat to the integrity of the self in chronic conditions. Basic assumptions about the self may have to be discarded as a response to the unexpected challenges forced upon the person. Having to use a wheelchair, for example, threatens the beliefs a person may have about being mobile. If you can no longer freely decide to go shopping, then your view of self may be radically altered by your loss of independence. Haggstrom, Axelsson and Norberg (1994) describe a qualitative study with 29 people who had suffered a stroke. Following analysis of interviews about their reactions to their condition, four main themes were found: uncertainty; sadness and mourning; gratefulness, hope and satisfaction; and isolation. Conrad (1987) identified major themes about the experience of chronic illness, and these included uncertainty in relation to obtaining the diagnosis and the uncertain future after the condition has been recognized. Also family relations were identified as extremely vulnerable in this context, as was the person's known self-concept and personal biography. The management of symptoms and medication was also defined by Conrad as a major theme running through the lives of all who suffered chronic illness. This also linked into difficulties with gaining information about the condition and finding ways of coping with it.

Christenson & Anderson (1989) showed in their survey that stroke with aphasia has a greater negative impact on the patient's spouse than does stroke without aphasia. For the spouses of aphasic patients sampled in this study, role changes represented the major adjustment made to the partner's stroke. These adjustments were greater than those experienced by partners of nonaphasic patients. This was explained by the fact that aphasic partners had more difficulty communicating about details concerned with role adjustments. However, both spouse groups were affected to some degree by communication problems associated with stroke and Christenson and Anderson record the importance of evaluating communication between the stroke patient (regardless of aphasia or not) and the spouse or partner.

In terms of meeting individual needs there has been considerably less work reported until recently. Brumfitt & Clarke (1983) described the application of psychotherapeutic approaches to the management of the aphasic person. Friedland & McColl (1987) studied patients during the first two years after a stroke and identified four aspects to social support which could provide positive and useful support. These were: a) satisfaction with social support; b) the single most significant relationship in the individual's life; c) close friends and family; and d) the community. Tanner and Gerstenberger (1988) discuss the dimensions of loss which occur following aphasic onset and recommend that treatment takes account of the grief response. Brumfitt (1989) discussed the recovery pattern of an aphasic person in a single case study which interprets the emotional recovery as a bereavement reaction. Williams (1996) discussed various approaches to therapy for stroke patients including the introduction of pet facilitated therapy, based on evidence from its effectiveness with other populations, such as psychiatric patients. Cognitive therapy is also recommended. Psychological support can be provided through many forms of group therapy, such as that reported by Rice *et al.* (1983) where information about stroke was part of the overall aim of the group as well as the provision of support.

It is suggested that other approaches to helping the stroke patient could be developed, as discussed below.

Personal Construct Theory

One way of looking at the aphasic person's predicament is to use the psychological model, Personal Construct Theory, developed by Kelly in the 1950s and subsequently applied to communication disorders by Fay Fransella in the 1960s.

Kelly (1955) developed Personal Construct Theory (PCT) as a way of describing how we understand ourselves and other people. His theory comes from social psychology and focuses on the importance of the individual's construct system. That is, in Kelly's terms, the way in which an individual understands the reality of his world is based upon the discriminations he learns and the predictions he makes about the future. Thus, a patient in hospital may base his understanding of the situation on his past knowledge of hospitals and his predictions about hospitals in general.

The fundamental philosophical assumption underlying Personal Construct Theory is constructive alternativism which asserts that, 'all of our present interpretations of the universe are subject to revision or replacement' (Kelly, 1955). Thus the belief that something is fact is instead viewed as a possible interpretation. The relevance of this for clinical work is clearly seen. The interpretation of the client's predicament by the clinician can be viewed in many ways, just as the interpretation by the client of his own predicament can be viewed in alternative ways. Construing is therefore an active process whereby we evaluate and give meaning to all aspects of life, rather like a scientist – making hypotheses, testing them out, and if necessary revising them on the basis of the evidence we collect. Constructs are bipolar, thus the individual makes choices about how an event may be construed. That is, meeting new people may be construed as exciting or challenging (according to one individual's construct system). Generally, in Kellian terminology, the events themselves are described as 'elements'.

What is important about this theory is that it emphasises the individual difference and offers explanations for why this should be. Useful descriptions of this theory can be seen in Fransella & Dalton, 1990; Dalton, 1994; and Winter, 1992.

The theoretical position of PCT

Personal Construct Theory can offer a theoretical perspective on the individual's predicament which can enhance our understanding and thus empower us therapeutically. There is no doubt that a major change is forced upon a person who suffers a stroke and that this change is manifested in the loss of all previous roles. Potentially, whatever the construct system was before the stroke, the individual patient may have to review his construing of everything in his life. What he might previously have construed as easy, he now may construe as difficult. For example, at first the individual is forced to take on the role of patient and subsequently on return from hospital may attempt to resume the roles that were part of the pre-illness state.

In personal construct terms, the change affects core role construing. Kelly defined core construing as the system of constructs which deal specifically with the self: that is, our most central and personal issues, as illustrated by the case study of Mrs V below.

Mrs V suffered a stroke and was left with a hemiplegia which meant she could no longer work in the cafe she shared with her husband, or look after her two-year-old grandson. Two of her major core roles were lost to her by becoming disabled. Her relationship with her husband was damaged because she could no longer be a workmate with her husband and her role of caretaker of her grandson. Thus the most important ways of functioning were now inaccessible to her.

This loss of important core roles may be catastrophic. The individual is forced to look at life from a different perspective. Not only has the individual lost current roles, but the individual has lost potential roles in the future. For example, Mrs V may be unable to help her husband expand the cafe into a larger development and thus miss the enjoyment of that shared experienced.

Kelly viewed the major disruption of core roles as a state of transition: that is, a process of reconstruing needs to take place if core roles have been seriously disrupted. There are four states which can be usefully applied to the predicament of the stroke patient:

- Guilt: awareness of dislodgement of the self from one's core structure.
- Threat: awareness of imminent comprehensive change in one's core structure.
- Anxiety: the recognition that the events with which one is confronted lie outside the range of convenience of one's construct system.
- Anger: awareness of invalidation of constructs leading to hostility.

Although guilt is often attributed to 'doing wrong', what Kelly importantly draws out is the experience of finding ourselves to be behaving 'differently'. So that while the stroke patient is forced to live a disabled life, he is forced out of his core roles and there is a strong experience of 'this is not like me'. That causes the feelings of guilt.

Threat may relate to the feature of realization in the bereavement process (Murray Parkes, 1978): that the recognition of self as a disabled person may be invalidating and that making sense of it all at first, is too difficult. So the person may need a significant amount of recovery time, in order to develop a new set of constructs which take account of the disability.

Anxiety is described by Kelly as a process whereby the individual somehow loses his 'structural grip' on his situation. At a simple level, if you are about to take an examination, you are unable to make predictions about the questions (although you have have a set of constructs which are to do with examinations in general). Thus, you become anxious. You cannot construe how you will be during the examination because you do not know what effect the question will have on you.

At the core role level, the individual who has suffered a stroke, finds many current roles to be invalid and thus experiences anxiety because he or she has no constructs about being a person with a disability. This anxiety may come in waves and relate to facing new experiences. For example, dealing with family may become possible quickly, but meeting new people as a disabled person may cause tremendous anxiety because the person has no constructs about behaving with strangers as a disabled person.

Anger is something frequently referred to in the grief model. It seems to relate to the same issue, which is that when the person finds their pre-illness constructs invalidated, instead of attempting to reconstrue, the response of anger occurs. This has been described as 'stalling for time when faced with invalidation'. Thus the individual can stay with the old construction of self, while searching for alternative ways of construing (Murray Parkes, 1975).

Using PCT in therapy

It is helpful to view adapting to a stroke as a process of transition. That is, the individual comes to understand and make sense of the personal situation by moving through phases of construing. Veny *et al.* (1989) evaluated therapy groups for elderly people using a Personal Construct Therapy approach. Following 12 weeks of therapy and when compared to a matched control group, the therapy group showed less anxiety, depression and indirectly expressed anger. More feelings of competence and well-being were also found.

There has been a long history of using Personal Construct Theory in the understanding and treatment of stuttering problems (Fransella, 1972). This has enabled the practising therapist to understand the condition more fully and thus enhance the effectiveness of the therapy. Indeed, Fransella's work was innovative in that it moved the understanding of stuttering away from the act of speaking and focused more fully on the implications of this condition for the individual. This approach is now well established in Britain (Hayhow & Levy, 1989), and some subsequent work followed this (Dalton, 1983; Levy, 1987).

Surprisingly, the knowledge gained from the application of Personal Construct Theory to stuttering has not been extensively applied to other communicative problems. Thus, the literature on stroke and aphasia is sparse. Brumfitt (1985) reported a study using repertory grid technique with two groups of aphasic people. The reaction to loss of communicative ability is also discussed in relation to the personal construct model. The results from the grids showed that all subjects construed their past selves as different from their present selves, and importantly, that their past selves were also construed as their ideal selves. It is suggested that the issue of searching for the lost self in the grief model is associated with this result. Dalton (1994) discusses joint counselling sessions with a couple where the husband was dysphasic. The way in which the couple were helped to resolve their difficulties was by specific focus on increasing the communication between the two. This was achieved by using drawing with the dysphasic person, who was asked to draw contrasting constructs about different aspects of his life. For example, he drew pictures of himself as 'OK' and 'not OK'. The drawings formed the basis for developing a conversation about issues which were of concern to him.

Cunningham (1998) in a recent study reported the process of counselling a severely aphasic speaker using Personal Construct Therapy. Sessions were patient led, but information from repertory grids was used to inform the sessions. Cunningham noted that the repertory grid procedure was a useful exercise which provided insight for the clinician and permitted the client an opportunity to talk about himself. Although it was difficult to demonstrate change after six sessions of Personal Construct Therapy, the report acknowledges the more positive construing of the client and a notable improvement in self-confidence as a communicator.

The construing processes of the aphasic person

Personal Construct Theory was devised primarily for people with intact language systems. Indeed, there is no mention in Kelly's original work about the application of the theory to communication disorders. This has obviously been a later application. Although the work on stuttering has been evolved as an extension of the original, there arises the question of the applicability of this theory to people with potential comprehension and expressive problems. Although PCT is often viewed as a verbal theory, because of the importance in eliciting verbal constructs, Kelly (1995) did write about preverbal and nonverbal construing.

Preverbal constructs

As Bannister and Fransella (1986) stated, 'a construct is not a verbal label'. Preverbal constructs refer to those constructs which have been developed before a child has language. An example of this would be comfort versus discomfort, hungry versus not hungry. Although we have no experimental data, it is conceivable that those preverbal constructs are intact even in the most handicapped aphasic person, and even if the person is unable to produce the verbal label for them.

Nonverbal constructs

This type of construing is often referred to in relation to sensory experience, such as drawing, appreciation of visual images, and listening to music. Dalton (1994) refers to a successful session with a disabled woman who listened to music with her husband, and thus they were reminded of their relationship before her illness. From these memories it was easier to develop a productive conversation.

Acquired brain damage

The most formal way of doing this was devised by Kelly (1955) and was originally called the Role Construct Repertory Test. Since then, various modifications have taken place to form the repertory grid technique in use today. The technique aims to elicit constructs from a person by asking them to consider groups of 'elements' or role titles which have been selected from their social context. The elements are written along the top of the grid, and the bipolar constructs are written down the side. Each element is considered in relation to each pair of constructs. It is important to note that the grid is not a test and as noted by Hayhow & Levy (1989), that both therapist and client are aware of why they are taking part in the exercise and what it is going to tell them.

Eliciting constructs

Using the traditional format, three 'roles', or people, as elements are initially considered. Elements are what people construe, and as Epting (1984) says, these can be anything from fur caps, mathematical symbols through to personal characteristics of self. In the elicitation procedure, the individual is then asked to consider 'whether two of the elements are alike in some important way that distinguishes them from the third' (Kelly, 1955). For our purposes here, we are using self-elements. The label which is elicited from this is described as the emergent pole of the construct. The individual is then asked to supply the opposite of the pole which has just been described. This label is the contrasting pole of the construct and is the implicit pole.

An example of the procedure would be that three elements are considered:

- Self before illness
- Self now
- Self I would like to be

The emergent pole of the construct which was elicited was 'self-confident'. The implicit pole was elicited in response to the emergent pole and was 'don't know self'.

Other forms of elicitation have been suggested where the previous type of triad method has seemed too complex. Supplied constructs can be used, and here the only requirement is that the individual be able to supply the constructs to the elements selected. Bannister and Fransella discuss the issue of supplied versus elicited constructs (1977). One of the criticisms of supplied constructs is that the structure of the grid becomes more like a questionnaire. However, there is no doubt that this may be the only approach to use with very disabled people, if the requirement is for a formal repertory grid. This has been used with people who have learning disabilities.

Brumfitt (unpublished work) used a series of photographs with severely impaired aphasic people which served as a stimulus for the production of the construct label. The grids which were produced were small, and the results limited because of this. An example of the constructs elicited from photographs was as follows:

- very good : very bad
- can move : can't move
- happy : sad
- angry : not angry
- starting life : finishing life

Brumfitt (1985) also used repertory grids with aphasic people who had a higher level of ability. A standard elicitation procedure was used. The constructs elicited were divided into themes, and three main strands were noted. Firstly, there were those which related to people's behaviour in relation to the aphasic – for example if they were patient or impatient. Secondly, constructs focused around achievement and being fulfilled. Finally, it was possible to distinguish a theme about communication and the ability to socialize.

An example from Brumfitt's study of constructs from a grid is presented below:

- short tempered : not short tempered
- very kind : not so kind

- calm : more excitable
- sense of humour : less sense of humour
- have purpose : no purpose
- have patients : not so much
- part of a team : work for yourself
- meticulous : not so meticulous
- listen to you : poor listener
- enjoys eating : does not enjoy eating

Both types of grid required the aphasic people to rate the different elements in relation to these constructs. This was a noticeably difficult task for people with problems in making semantic distinctions and retaining language while completing a task. There are ways of simplifying the procedure. For example, instead of asking the person to rate each element on each construct dimension, it is easier to ask them to rank the elements in order of closeness to each construct dimension. An example of this is given by the case study of Mr A who with the construct pair 'outgoing versus shy' ranked each element in relation to how near it was to the emergent pole of 'being outgoing':

- Past self
- Wife
- Work colleague
- Son
- Ideal self
- A person I feel sorry for
- How I expect I'll be in the future

Thus, Mr A's past self is rated as most outgoing, and his construction of himself in the future is rated as least outgoing. The rating number can then be applied to the elements by the therapist in discussion with the client. Hayhow and Levy (1987) suggest that the presentation of a single element with a list of constructs may also be useful in helping people make distinctions. Again this simplifies the task.

It is important to note that the grid also serves as a significant conversation in itself. Completing the grid allows the client to have an overview of his own psychological world and understand himself in ways which were previously inaccessible. Often, just the process of doing it may give important insights.

Analysis of the grid

When a grid is complete, a matrix of numbers will indicate the rating of the elements in relation to the constructs. In the first instance it is useful to look over the material without formal analysis. This will give some indication of which elements are construed similarly, for example. The distance between elements is of great interest, and this can be covered in the computational analysis of the grid. However, the specific issue is whether certain elements are viewed as close or distant from each other. Past-self and present-self may be shown to be significantly far apart which would then form a basis for therapeutic intervention. Another concern relates to the amount of variance taken out by the first component when the grid is formally analysed: that is, if a substantial amount of construing process is accounted for in the first component, it gives an indication of how much those particular constructs are used for making sense of the world. Formal understanding of the grid can be achieved by computer analysis (Beail, 1985; and Bannister and Fransella, 1977) which can give information about the clustering of constructs, the element distances, the significant relationships between the constructs and the amount of structure in the grid. Some examples of computer programmes are INGRID (Slater, 1977), GAB (Bannister and Higginbotham, 1983), and GRAN (1988).

Self-characterization

Kelly devised this as another way of finding out about how the individual views his or her life role. Many accounts of this can be found (Kelly, 1955; Epting, 1984; Hayhow & Levy, 1989; Winter, 1992). The instructions from Kelly's original work are:

> 'I want you to write a character sketch of . . . , just as if he/she were a principal character in a play. Write it as it might be written by a friend who knew him/her very intimately and very sympathetically, perhaps better than anyone ever really could know him/her. Be sure to write it in the third person. For example, start out by saying
> . . . . is . . . . '

It is suggested that individuals may find it easier to describe themselves in writing. Of course this may not always be the case with the stroke patient who may find this task much more difficult, but there is a strong argument for the value of being able to sit privately and write and reflect on self. As with people with language disability who would have difficulty with this type of task, it is possible to simplify this in the way suggested by Jackson and Bannister (1985) where the therapist acts as secretary and writes down for the client. An example of a self-characterization completed with an aphasic person is given below:

> 'X is OK now. Stroke long time now, got used to it. Don't bother me. Nice flat, can manage OK. Before sporty, not now. Er, go and watch, help out. Nice time. Still get fed up, bored, no job. Try to help people.'

Even with this restricted type of characterization, it is possible to get an understanding of the individual constructs which are important. Kelly (1955) describes the analysis which is intended to bring the individual's construing into a focus.

Firstly, the clinician should consider the sequences and transitions that the characterization reveals, then the organization of the protocol looking for topic sentences. In particular, Kelly advises the clinician to look at opening sentences which may give an indication of the issue which could be the 'safest ground' to begin therapy from. Kelly notes that there are several different approaches to writing a self-characterization. There is the 'personal record approach': name, age and sex and so on. There is what Kelly terms the 'outside to inside' approach which goes from superficial appearance to inner reality; and there is the 'problem' approach which begins with a statement of the key problem which the client sees himself as facing.

An example of this approach is the use of an opening sentence such as: 'Mary just can't seem to stay friends with anyone for long.' Here the opening sentence reveals the 'problem' approach where Mary has enough insight to be able to identify what her difficulties are, even though she may not be able to solve them.

Kelly also suggests that the analysis is concerned with 'reflection against context': that is, the clinician takes each statement and considers it not only as an independent statement but also as what it might mean in the context of the characterization as a whole.

In addition, the clinician is advised to be aware of the repetition of terms, as in the example quoted below where the use of 'frightened child' as an explanation for herself is repeated by Katy. In therapy the clinician would need to explore that construct with her.

'Katy is just like a frightened child when she has to meet new people. She feels they will notice that her arm is paralysed and that she is not an attractive person. This frightened child person always shrinks into her shell and can't make small talk. If Katy wasn't a frightened child, it would be easier to get on with life.'

As Winter (1992) notes, the self-characterization forms the basis for enabling the clinician to understand the client's construing and can also be used in other ways: for example, to know what the client's future goals and hopes are. A self-characterization can be used for this by asking the individual to write about himself in five years' time. Alternatively, it may be useful to know how the client construes himself in the past; thus, self five years before or self as a child could be considered. All of these approaches can be used to build up understanding and enable the clinician to use the therapy time more relevantly.

Therapists who use repertory grids or self-characterizations gain a good understanding about how the world is viewed by the individual. This may be of crucial importance when helping someone who has a long life history before coming to therapy. It also clarifies what meaning the difficulties have for the individual.

The therapeutic approach

A very useful description of therapy can be found in Epting (1984), but this is not specific to people who have suffered strokes. However, the process that Epting describes is applicable and relevant. A way of looking at helping someone cope with their disability is by thinking in terms of enabling the client to reconstrue. Kelly (1955) discusses the meaning of psychotherapeutic movement in this way.

(1)   the client has reconstrued himself and certain other features of his world within an original system;
(2)   he has organized his old system more precisely;
(3)   he has replaced some of the constructs in his old system with new ones.'

It would seem that this is what we are aiming for in the recovery process of the person who has suffered a stroke. Because of the effect on core roles, it is necessary for the client to do all of the types of reconstruction suggested by Kelly. Another way of describing this is to talk about elaborating a new sense of self, so that the individual is able to keep enough of the past self intact, but can evolve a new construction of post-stroke self which is positive and has stability and consistency.

With an acquired problem, there are several stages which form a necessary part of coping or recovery. It may be that some people move through these phases naturally as progress through physiotherapy, occupational and speech and language therapy occurs. Others may need to spend time evaluating their position. The stages below may occur over a very long period of time, such as over the first two years.

(1)   Working out with the client what meaning the loss of speech has. How are the disabilities construed in the individual's social context? Making sure that the construction of this is acknowledged.
(2)   Developing new constructs which allow the individual space and time to move from the acute to the long-term phase (these may or may not be temporary depending on the recovery potential of the person).
(3)   Establishing self-constructs which the individual finds acceptable and allow opportunities for further development.

Of course, the development of new constructs is not a passive event. This is intrinsically related to behaviour. Often, the tasks set in therapy allow the person to reconstrue. For example, deciding to use the telephone again six months after the stroke may allow a construction of self as 'more independent'. What is important is that time is spent in discussing the implications of this success in terms of how this reconstruction works for the person.

In the example set out below, the client offers construct labels about how he sees himself since his stroke.

Therapist: 'How have things been this week?'
Client: 'Well, it's been, you know, hard, hard with her.'
Therapist: 'Do you mean your wife?'
Client: 'Yes. Em getting fed up.'
Therapist: 'In what way?'
Client: 'Me, me. Slow and stupid.'
Therapist: 'Do you think she feels you are slow and stupid?'
Client: 'Yes, yes. Before, drive her around, shopping, buy nice things.'
Therapist: 'So, the way you are now is different from before?'
Client: 'Yes, before OK. Now no good.'

Slow, stupid and no good are offered as one side of the construct pairs. Clearly, the client is making the distinction between his past and current self, but is also using as a marker the way he construes his wife construing him. It may not be the case that his wife views him in this way, but the important issue here is that the client at this moment believes it to be the reality of the situation. As he appears to be using his belief about his wife's view of him to define himself, this would need to be explored further in therapy because of the effect this would have on his recovery.

As with many counselling approaches, it is important to use the language of the client; and is particularly so in Personal Construct Theory. The language chosen by the client represents the way the individual construes, and the therapist has to stay in that context in order to help the process move on.

In the case set out below, John talks about his distress at his changed ability in talking:

'I know I talk slowly than what I could do before the stroke, but, er, it was a shock, because round here people talk quick and I talked quicker than them and I miss the words out, the little words and that. I think it was a shock.'

Note the use of the contrast between before his stroke and afterwards. It is important to acknowledge the pain caused by the loss of his abilities. This seems to relate to the same issue as searching for the lost self, as discussed in bereavement reactions (Murray Parkes, 1975). Time spent acknowledging the loss can be positive for the client. This may involve a very concrete discussion about the way the individual used to be. For example, John used to bring in certificates of his qualifications as a laboratory technician and wanted to talk about his job and his contribution to his place of work. This was viewed as necessary to helping the process of reconstrual, because in 'reliving' his past he was able to begin to leave it behind and move on to the future. Encouraging discussion about construing future self is a way of moving on, but only when the client seems ready. Deciding when to do this needs clinical judgement.

Later, John talks about ways of coping and his feelings about himself.

Therapist: 'What words would you want to describe yourself before you came to the group?'

Client: 'Get frustrated a lot and bad tempered. But, er, normal I think, er, got a barrier up against the stroke. I make fun of myself I don't let anybody else get the first word in and that, er, I can look after myself if they are making fun of me.'

In spite of the language difficulty, this client has ability to self-ascribe and get his meaning across well. In this extract, he notes his negative feelings and can express them, but he also describes coping strategies, which indicate a positive strength in his development since his stroke.

Finally, John is able to acknowledge his position at a later stage.

'It's passing the time, er, now I can help out over there. Er, in the shop it's feeling better. I can do it. It's not like before, but OK, er, enjoy myself.'

Even in this small extract, it is possible to see the important constructs. For example, there is 'helping out', 'feeling better', 'can do', 'not like before' and 'enjoy myself'.

Conclusion

The application of Personal Construct Theory to our understanding of the reactions to stroke and acquired communication problems can offer theoretical insights which make it easier to understand the meaning of the problem to the individual and to understand the process the individual experiences in terms of emotional reactions. The use of repertory grid technique and self-characterization can offer a basic starting point for helping the person. Finally, as an approach to counselling, it offers a structure to the recovery process which aids our therapeutic understanding and can only benefit our clients.

References

Bannister, D. & Fransella, F. (1977) *A Manual for Repertory Grid Technique.* Academic Press, London.

Bannister, D. & Fransella, F. (1986) *Inquiring Man; The Psychology of Personal Constructs.* Croom Helm, London.

Bannister, D. & Higginbotham, P.G. (1983) *The GAB Computer Program for the Analysis of Repertory Grid Data.* Croom Helm, London.

Beail, N. (1985) *Repertory Grid Technique and Personal Constructs.* Croom Helm, London.

Blackman, N. (1950) Group psychotherapy with aphasics. *J. of Nervous & Mental Diseases* **3**, 154–63.

Brumfitt, S.M. & Clarke, P.R.F. (1983) An application of psychotherapeutic techniques to the management of aphasia. In *Aphasia Therapy*. (C. Code & D. Muller, eds), pp. 89–101. Arnold, London.

Brumfitt, S.M. (1985) The use of repertory grids with aphasic people. In *Repertory Grid Technique and Personal Constructs*. (N. Beail, ed). Croom Helm, London.

Brumfitt, S.M. (1989) A psychosocial case discussion. *Proceedings of the British Aphasiology Conference*. Cambridge, England.

Bury, M.R. (1982) Chronic illness as biographical disruption. *Sociology of Health and Illness* **4**, 167–82.

Christenson, J.M. & Anderson, J.D. (1989) Spouse adjustment to stroke: aphasic versus nonaphasic partners. *J. Commun. Disord.* **22**, 225–231.

Code, C. & Muller, D. (1993) *The Code Muller Protocols; Assessing Perceptions of Psychosocial Adjustment to Aphasia and Related Disorders*. Whurr Publications, London.

Conrad, P. (1987) The experience of illness; recent and new directions in the experience and management of chronic illness. In *Research in the sociology of health care* **6**, JAI Press, Greenwich CT.

Cunningham, R. (1998) Counselling someone with severe aphasia: an explorative case study. *Disability and Rehabilitation* **20**(9), 346–54.

Dalton, P. (1983) *Approaches to the Treatment of Stuttering*. Croom Helm, London.

Dalton, P. (1994) *Counselling People with Communication Problems*. Sage Publications, London.

Epting, F. (1984) *Personal Construct Counselling and Psychotherapy*. John Wiley, Chichester.

Fransella, F. (1972) *Personal Change and Reconstruction*. Academic Press, London.

Fransella, F. & Dalton, P. (1990) *Personal Construct Counselling in Action*. Sage Publications, London.

Friedland, J. & McColl, M.A. (1987) Social support and psychosocial dysfunction after stroke; buffering effects in a community sample. *Archives of Physical Medicine and Rehabilitation* **68**, 475–480.

Haggstrom, T., Axelstson, K. & Norberg, A. (1994) The experience of living with stroke sequelae illuminated by means of stories and metaphors. *Qualitative Health Research* **4**(3), 321–337.

Hayhow, R. & Levy, C. (1989) *Working with Stuttering*. Winslow Press, Oxon.

Kelly, G. (1955) *The Psychology of Personal Constructs*. Vols 1 & 2. W.W. Norton, New York.

Jackson, S. & Bannister, D. (unpublished paper) referred to in *Working with Stuttering* (R. Hayhow & C. Levy, eds). Winslow Press, Oxon.

Leach, C. (1988) GRAN: A computer program for the cluster analysis of a repertory grid. *Br. J. of Clinical Psychology* **27**, 173–4.

Levy, C. (1987) Interiorised stuttering; a group therapy approach. In *Stuttering Therapy; Practical Approaches*. Croom Helm, London.

Mulley, G.T. (1985) *Practical Management of Stroke*. Croom Helm, London.

Murray Parkes, C. (1975) *Bereavement*. Pelican Books, England.

Niemi, M.L., Laaksonen, M.A., Kotila, M.D. & Waltimo, O. (1988) Quality of life four years after stroke. *Stroke* **19**(9), 1101–07.

Redinger, R.A., Forster, S., Dolphin, M.K., Godduhn, J. & Weisinger, J. (1971) Group therapy in the rehabilitation of the severely aphasic and hemiplegic in the late stages. *Scand. J. of Rehab. Med.* **3**(1), 89–91.

Rice, B., Paull, A. & Muller, D. (1983) An evaluation of a social support group for spouses and aphasic adults. *Aphasiology* **3**, 247–256.

Robinson, R.G., Bolduc, P.L. & Price, T.R. (1987) Two-year longitudinal study of post stroke mood disorders: diagnosis and outcome at one and two years. *Stroke* **18**, 837–43.

Rollin, W. (1987) *The Psychology of Communication Disorders in Individuals and Their Families.* Prentice Hall, New Jersey.

Royal College of Speech and Language Therapists (1991) *Communicating Quality; Professional Standards for Speech and Language Therapists*, London.

Slater, P. (ed.) (1977) *The Measurement of Interpersonal Space by Grid Technique*, Vol. 2. John Wiley, London.

Tanner, D. & Gerstenberger, D.L. (1988) The grief response in neuropathologies in speech and language. *Aphasiology* **2**, 79–84.

Veny, L.L., Benjamin, Y.N. & Preston, C.A. (1989) An evaluation of personal construct therapy for the elderly. *Br. J. of Medical Psychology* **62**, 35–41.

Warhborg, P. & Borenstein, P. (1989) Family therapy in families with an aphasic family member. *Aphasiology* **3**, 93–7.

Williams, S.E. (1996) Psychological adjustment following stroke. In *Adult Aphasia Rehabilitation* (G.L. Wallace, ed.). Butterworth Heineman Publishers, Boston.

Winter, D. (1992) *Personal Construct Psychology in Clinical Practice.* Routledge, London.

Chapter 11

Everyday Problems of Daily Living

Avril Drummond

The role of the occupational therapist

Occupational therapists (known as OTs) have much to offer the patient with a stroke and their carers. They assess everyone as an individual, consider the particular problems and difficulties experienced by each patient and carer and offer advice, treatment and practical help. Thus the aim of occupational therapy is to help each patient achieve the highest level of independence and ability possible (Stroke Association, 1992).

A large proportion of the OT professional training involves studying the psychological aspects of illness. OTs are therefore aware of the emotional effects of stroke and understand the difficulties which patients face afterwards such as memory problems, feeling depressed, and problems in controlling emotions. OTs can provide reassurance to the patient and carer, give advice, and offer support.

An important part of the work of the OT is re-educating patients in activities of daily living (ADL). Hopson (1981) has defined ADL as 'those tasks which all of us undertake every day of our lives in order to maintain our personal levels of care' – a rather grand title for everyday activities such as eating, washing and dressing. Patients may be referred for treatment when they are in hospital. Initially they will be seen on the ward and given advice on positioning and transferring from bed to chair. Early on they will also be given practice in activities such as getting washed and dressed. As patients improve, they will be assessed by the occupational therapy department for simple domestic chores such as preparing a hot snack and for advice on other activities such as getting in and our of the bath. In many instances the OT will accompany the patient home on a visit to check if any special equipment or adaptations are needed to make it easier to cope at home. The OT will teach the patient and carer how to use any equipment and adaptations provided. If the patient is not referred to the occupational therapy services while in hospital or is not admitted to hospital, a visit may be requested from a social services OT who works in the community and can also assess the patient and provide necessary aids and adaptations to the home.

ADL treatment is thus a vital aspect of rehabilitation, as most people want to be as independent as possible and not have to rely on others for help – particularly with basic self-care. Patients may be able to relearn skills through practice or find new ways of carrying out activities. It is, however, essential to realize that advice and ideas will not generalize to each patient's unique problems, circumstances and home environment. The OT needs to assess each individual and treat accordingly.

Although it has been demonstrated that the most extensively used goal in OT treatment is achieving personal independence (Andrews, 1984; Smith, 1989), patients may also be seen for other specific treatments. Superficially it may look as if patients are playing games or doing activities just to be kept amused. However, the activities given to patients meet specific treatment aims. For example, a game to improve a particular movement in the affected arm; woodwork to improve standing ability or to increase stamina; an activity to replace a hobby which the patient may no longer be able to do. Activities given by the occupational therapist are always purposeful; patients are not given activities just to fill in time. The word 'occupational' does not imply 'occupying' but 'occupation' – meaning work. Such activities are an important part of occupational therapy treatment, but they will not be construed further in this chapter which concentrates on everyday ADL problems.

Everyday problems of daily living

There are many areas which must be considered in the rehabilitation programme of the patient who has had a stroke. These everyday problems, which are predominantly dealt with by occupational therapists, will be considered under the following headings: home environment, eating, washing, personal care, toiletting, dressing, cooking and domestic tasks, getting around outside, leisure activities, general advice for carers.

The home environment

It is vital to consider accommodation. If the patient's home environment is not suitable, or cannot be made suitable, alternative arrangements may need to be made in the short term. It is important to consider four aspects: namely, access, the layout of the house, the layout of individual rooms, and furniture.

Access

Good access to the home is vital; otherwise, there will be problems getting in and out of the house. Even if the person does not want to go out for specific reasons, such as visiting friends or going to the shops, it is important that he/she is able to go outdoors. It is also vital that someone can get out of the home in the event of a fire or similar emergency.

If the person who has suffered a stroke is in a wheelchair, paths may need to be ramped. However, care is needed to ensure that the gradient of ramps is not too steep. There is no benefit in replacing steep steps with an equally steep slope! It is better initially to use portable ramps before having concrete ones built; if the patient makes a good recovery and is eventually able to walk, a ramp may prove more of a problem than steps. It is usual to wait approximately six months after a stroke before making major permanent alterations to access.

If the patient is ambulant, grab rails can be fitted beside steps or along paths. If steps are very steep, it may be possible to build additional steps between to make them easier to climb.

Layout

The general layout of the accommodation needs to be considered. If the stroke sufferer is unable to manage stairs, it may be necessary to bring the bed downstairs and for the patient to wash at the kitchen sink and use a commode. As a long-term solution it may be appropriate to consider having a downstairs extension built on to the home. If this is a serious consideration, the social services OT can give advice on planning the actual extension, as well as providing important information on grants and eligibility for funding. If the patient lives in council accommodation, it may be worthwhile investigating the possibility of a housing transfer.

If the patient has to use the stairs because of cramped conditions or personal preference, a second stair rail may be needed which ensures that there is always a rail to hold with the non-affected arm. It is a good idea to limit the number of times the person goes upstairs initially; for example, some individuals only go up the stairs to bed at night and come down in the morning. During the day a commode, bottle, or downstairs toilet can be used. If the patient is unable to climb the stairs but needs to do so, the installation of a stair lift may be appropriate as a long-term solution.

Individual rooms

Whether someone is in a wheelchair or ambulant, highly polished floors are to be avoided for obvious reasons. Rugs and mats should also be lifted, as it is easy to catch the toes of the affected leg when concentrating on walking. Loose rugs are also awkward to negotiate by those in a wheelchair, as they have a tendency to fold up and lock in the wheels.

A room with a lot of furniture may be useful to someone with an unsteady walk who can 'furniture walk'. However, furniture can present an obstacle course for someone who uses a walking frame or a wheelchair and needs to be able to move through doorways and have space to turn. Consequently, individual rooms should be tailored to mobility needs.

Rails may be needed in specific rooms in the house, such as the toilet and bathroom, for safety and ease of transfer. The OT can give advice on rails and arrange for them to be fitted. However, because of the length of waiting lists in many areas for fitting, many carers just want advice on the type of rail to fit and where to position it on the wall. Grab rails should never be fitted on plaster board walls.

Consideration also needs to be given to heating. Many people who have had a stroke complain that they are more sensitive to the cold, so it is important that heating is adequate. Patients who sit for long periods often need a blanket around their feet. Direct heat on the affected side should be avoided – particularly if the person has reduced sensation.

Furniture

Many patients and carers make the mistake of going out to buy a new chair or bed as soon as a stroke is diagnosed. However, this is not always necessary, as existing furniture can be modified or borrowed from social services or the Red Cross for an interim period.

The height of furniture is important for ease of transfer; it is very difficult to get onto and up from a bed or chair which is very low. Furniture can be raised to the height required by putting bed blocks and chair blocks under the legs which are designed with safety features. Well-meaning relatives and friends may insert pieces of wood to increase the height of furniture; but if the patient is unsteady, there is real potential for an accident.

In the long term, if patients want to buy a more suitable bed or chair, it is possible to arrange a visit to a local Disabled Living Centre where they will get independent advice and have the opportunity to try out equipment. If patients decide to buy direct from a shop, they should be advised not to be impressed by medical sounding labels on products (for example, 'ortho-') which suggest they have additional benefits. For those who have great problems in getting up from a chair, it is possible to get electric and manual ejector chairs which help push the person to standing.

When purchasing a chair, there are several points to bear in mind:

- the back should be straight, not sloping, and support the back;
- the actual seat should be firm and high: knees should be bent at approximately 90°;
- armrests should be long and at a height where they can be used to push-up from more easily;
- the chair should be comfortable and stable;
- the seat covering should be considered carefully if the patient has problems with continence.

When buying a bed, the following should be considered:

- the mattress should be neither too hard nor too soft;
- the patient should be able to sit on the bed with their feet flat on the floor and without their knees bending excessively;
- does the patient want to buy a single or a double bed? If he/she has been used to sleeping in a double bed with someone, there is no obvious reason why this should not continue – unless both have made a conscious decision otherwise;
- avoid purchasing a hospital type bed which has an overhead pole for the patient to lever up on. This encourages over-use of the non-affected side and may increase the spasticity in the affected side. However, when in doubt, individual situations should be discussed with the therapist involved.

Eating

Individuals who have had a stroke may have problems eating for a variety of reasons:

- Difficulty swallowing because of poor head control or poor sitting position. Any patient who has swallowing problems should be referred for a full assessment;
- Problems chewing food because of poor sensation in one side of the face, or poor movement in the facial muscles and the tongue. If one side of the face is asymmetrical due to paralysis, it may be uncomfortable to wear dentures, and this obviously compounds the problem of chewing;
- Drinking can be a great problem, as it is more difficult to control liquid than food;
- Difficulty using cutlery because of poor movement or no movement in one hand;
- Difficulty keeping the plate or bowl steady for the same reason, which results in 'chasing' food around;
- Food gets cold because it takes a long time to eat and is therefore unappetising;
- Spilling food or dribbling; the embarrassment caused makes eating on social occasions a major problem for some patients;
- Visual and perceptual problems may result in not seeing food on the table or misjudging distances.

Solutions

Meal times should be unhurried and relaxed. The patient should sit in a good posture with the head supported in an upright position if necessary. Never position someone so that the head is tilted back, as this may make them choke. The affected side of the body, particularly the arm, should be positioned carefully.

As a general rule, patients should only be assisted when it is necessary – for example, if food is difficult to cut up – as it is a great morale boost to feed yourself. Eating is also a very personal activity, and people choose to eat their food in different ways. For example, some individuals like to eat their vegetables first and leave their meat until the end; some like to mix all the food together; others like to stop and rest in the middle of a course. If you are being fed by someone else, you are unable to exercise all your own idiosyncrasies and, consequently, the meal is not as enjoyable. It is therefore important that patients feed themselves as soon as possible.

Also:

- If the patient takes a long time to eat, it is best to serve small portions and keep food warm. Otherwise, specially insulated plates can be purchased.
- Do not put another course out until the present course is finished. This tends to pressurize the patient and emphasize the fact that they eat slowly.
- Do not replace forks with spoons – if someone can eat with a spoon, they can usually use a fork. It can be very degrading to eat a main course with a spoon.
- If someone can drink from a beaker, they can usually use an ordinary cup. Many patients complain that the majority of nursing beakers resemble those beakers provided for toddlers.
- Straws can be used to improve poor lip control. They are also easily transportable, and socially acceptable.
- Never fill a cup or mug too full of liquid, and always check that it is not too hot.
- Napkins or serviettes should be used in preference to towels to collect spills.
- If the patient persistently leaves food on the plate, check that he/she intended to do this – not that they are missing it because of visual or perceptual problems.
- Patients who have problems with chewing because of ill-fitting dentures should be referred urgently to a dentist.
- If the patient has sensory loss in the face, it is important to check that no food has been left in that side of the mouth (in the cheek) after mealtimes. This is important if individuals are in the habit of lying down after dinner, as this can lead to choking.
- Special eating aids are available for those with specific problems. Several companies manufacture special aids which can be used one-handed, such as a combined fork and knife, a combined spoon and fork, and special 'rocking' knives which make cutting easier. Adhesive place mats prevent plates and bowls moving around while cutting or putting food onto cutlery.
- Plate guards are devices which clip onto plates and stop food falling over the edge. They also provide a 'buffer' against which one can lever food onto the fork. Some companies market special plates with built-in lips which can be used in the same way. Plates can be purchased which belong to particular sets of china (for example, Royal Doulton), and this means that the individual who has some problems in eating can blend in on social occasions.
- Built-up handles on cutlery can be used where someone has movement in

their hemiplegic side. This may improve the grip and enable both hands to be used. However, note that handles should be lightweight – there is no point in providing cutlery with large handles which are too heavy to be lifted easily.

- Finally, remember that there is a danger of the immobile or less mobile patient with a stroke putting on weight. Although it may seem cruel, calorie intake may need to be reduced. The stroke patient who is overweight has many additional problems to contend with, especially if they already need help in moving around. Seek dietary advice if necessary and encourage carers to plan menus carefully. Some patients become constipated because of the combination of a poor diet and little exercise, and it is therefore vital that roughage is included in the diet.

Washing

Washing – at a sink, wash basin, in the bath or in a shower – is important not only for reasons of hygiene, but also for self-esteem. Patients who are immobile, or less mobile, often complain of feeling uncomfortable, and complain that they perspire more. The hemiplegic hand particularly can smell offensive if not washed regularly. Patients have problems washing because of lack of movement in one side, poor balance, diminished sensation, lack of energy, visual and perceptual problems.

General principles:

- It is important to test the temperature of water before washing or bathing someone. If the patient checks the temperature, make sure they do it with their non-affected hand. Cold water should be put in the bath first.
- It may be easier for the patient to use liquid soap or soap on a rope.
- Some patients prefer using a sponge rather than a flannel, as it is easier to manoeuvre and control. A wash mitt (a flannel in the shape of a glove) may also be easier to use with only one hand.
- Encourage patients to use their affected hand and arm as much as possible. Even if they have no real movement in the arm, it can still be used as a prop; for example, the flannel can be laid over the affected arm and soap applied by the other hand.
- Applying talc to the skin after drying soaks up residual moisture and, of course, makes it smell pleasant (although prolonged use may dry out the skin). Be careful of sticky creams and lotions in hot weather which makes the skin damp and greasy.
- Unless the individual with a stroke has an excellent recovery, they will probably need some physical assistance with washing their feet, under their unaffected arm and their back.
- Sewing loops on the ends of towels may make them more manageable for the patient to use. One end of the towel can then be 'anchored' in a fixed position, while the non-affected hand moves the towel around.

At the wash basin

It is best to use a seat rather than attempting to get the patient to stand for long periods and becoming fatigued. Use a chair which will not be damaged if it becomes wet. If the seat has a plastic surface, a towel may make it more comfortable to sit on. Where patients have problems with sensation, care is needed with positioning: for example, the hemiplegic leg should not come into contact with pipes under the wash basin.

At home, some carers find it easy to wash the patient after positioning him/her on a toilet. However, the problem with doing this is that the patient tends to take little part in the activity and has no opportunity of finding out how they are getting on from a mirror. Since they are usually pointing away from the wash basin, participation is not encouraged: consequently, this should be avoided if at all possible. Wash the top half of the person's body first and dry it completely – the patient should do as much as they are able, and, if necessary, have short rests. Do the bottom half next and again get the patient to do as much as possible. When standing to wash the bottom, try to wash and dry during one stand. If the patient needs help to stand, a rail may be needed at the side of the wash basin. Discourage the use of basins for leaning on; they were not designed for this purpose and can be pulled away from the wall over a period of time.

Bathing

Having a bath is more than just a way of keeping clean – it is relaxing and refreshing, and the psychological effects of soaking in the tub should not be underestimated. Nevertheless, safety is important and, if there is concern about getting someone in and out of the bath, strip washing should be encouraged. Incidentally, it is usually easy to get someone into a bath – the problem is always getting them out! Consider the size of the bathroom and whether there is enough room to transfer the patient. Consider whether there are enough safe, stable surfaces available to hold on to.

- As a rule of thumb, do not attempt to transfer someone in and out of a bath if you are in doubt that you can manage this.
- Try a dry run (that is, a bath with no water) with others available to help should the need arise.
- Avoid using bath oils which make baths (and patients!) slippery.
- **Always** use a non-slip mat.
- Consider putting grab rails on the walls. Ensure that the wall is solid and able to support both the rail and the weight of someone using it. Do not let patients use towel rails for this purpose – they are not designed to take the weight of someone.
- Special equipment, such as bath boards and bath seats, can be used to help transfer someone into the bath. The bath board lies across the bath, the

patient sits on it and swings the legs into the bath. The patient can then be lowered down onto the bath seat or remain on the board. Bath hoists can also be used to transfer the patient into the bath, although a full assessment from an occupational therapist is recommended before these are used.

• Bathing assistants to help with bathing are available in some areas.

Showers

It is essential that showers are thermostatically controlled so that the patient is not burnt. A shower may be used over a bath. Some carers position the patient on a bath board and use a shower attachment on the bathtaps to wash them down. Other carers use a conventional shower, and shower seats may be used so that the patient does not have to stand for long periods. Consider the access to the shower. For instance, a steep step into the shower may provide a serious obstacle to washing.

Personal care

NAILS: these need to be short and most patients need help to achieve this; clippers can be easier to use than scissors. Remember that nails are always more easily cut after the foot or hand has been soaked in warm water, but check the temperature of the water carefully. Suction nail brushes can be purchased to enable patients to clean their own nails. Most areas have a chiropodist who can advise on foot care.

SHAVING: If patients have facial sensation problems, it is best to encourage the use of an electric shaver. Remember to provide a mirror so that they can see what they are doing – unless they have perceptual problems, in which case a mirror may make the task more difficult.

TEETH: Tube dispensers are easier for patients to use than ordinary tubes of toothpaste. The patient may need to use their unaffected hand to clean their teeth, *but* they should still use their other hand as much as possible. Dentures can be soaked in the normal way.

MAKEUP: Wearing makeup can be a great morale boost, so encourage ladies to wear it if they normally use it. If the patient has movement in their hemiplegic hand but a poor grip, brush handles can be padded to make them bigger and consequently easier to use.

HAIR: Patients are likely to need help with washing and blow drying hair. A regular visit to the hairdresser can do more for self-confidence than can be imagined.

Toileting

Many patients and carers are embarrassed to ask for help with the problem of continence. Common problems which patients and their carers complain of include infections; urgency; frequency; physical problems in getting to the toilet; difficulty in manipulating clothes at the toilet; problems in getting onto the toilet.

General advice:

- Involve the consultant or GP if an infection or other medical problem is suspected.
- For male patients consider using a bottle, which can be kept close at hand.
- A commode can be used during the day and/or at night when it is often more difficult to get to the toilet. At home, commodes can be borrowed from the Red Cross and social services. They can be disguised as another chair in a bed sitting room if the patient feels embarrassed.
- Back fastening garments can be worn by those who need to have clothes removed quickly. Velcro can be used instead of buttons.
- Grab rails beside the toilet may assist transfers.
- If the toilet is low, a raised toilet seat can be provided – this will increase the height of the toilet by several inches and will mean that the patient does not have to bend so much.
- A regular routine of toileting for those who are incontinent is essential.
- If the toilet door opens inwards, the door may need to be re-hung. It is very difficult to get to someone who has fallen across the door and is blocking the access.
- Incontinence pads and plastic sheeting may be available from nursing services in some areas. Carers should be advised not to use sanitary towels instead of incontinence pads – they were not designed for this purpose and their use can lead to skin problems.
- Rolls of toilet paper can be awkward for patients with a stroke to manipulate one-handed; sheets of paper or wet wipe sheets are easier to manage.
- Contact and involve the nurse who specializes in continence advice about the provision of pads and any local laundry service.
- Patients with long-term problems may need to use a catheter.
- Monitor skin condition.
- As a long-term solution, it may be worthwhile to consider building an extension in a house which only has one toilet upstairs.

In addition to problems with continence, patients can also have problems with constipation, so it is important that roughage is included in the diet. However, medical advice should be sought if problems persist.

Dressing

Dressing is one of those tasks which we all take for granted, not only for warmth and comfort but for self-esteem and self-expression as well. Hospitals today recognize the importance of getting dressed and encourage patients to have their own clothes brought in so that they can get dressed as soon as possible.

However, it is known that many patients leave hospital without being able to dress themselves independently. Ebrahim & Nouri (1987) reported that 54% of patients in their study needed help with dressing six months after stroke. Recent research has demonstrated that it is possible to get such patients to improve their dressing performance (Walker *et al.*, 1996).

There are many reasons why people with a stroke have problems getting dressed and undressed. Difficulties occur because of problems with balance, visual problems, perceptual problems, poor concentration, difficulties manipulating clothes, and reduced stamina. Walker & Lincoln (1991) concluded in their study of dressing problems that 'the ability of the stroke patient to dress is heavily overshadowed by their physical disabilities.'

General advice:

- Undressing and dressing should be done in a warm, comfortable environment, as concentration is impossible when it is cold. If someone takes a long time to get dressed, make sure they are never sitting naked – put a towel or blanket around the lower half of their body to keep them warm and modest.
- Privacy is important.
- Try not to rush; take time and rest the patient as often as necessary – particularly when they are contributing to the task. Where this is not possible, for example, when patients have an early hospital appointment, it is important not to get flustered and agitated; this always makes the situation worse.
- Encourage the patient to sit as much as possible if they have problems with their balance. In hospital the OT may get patients to dress while sitting on the bed to improve their balance; at home carers should encourage them to sit in a chair.
- If clothes are positioned on the patient's affected side, it reinforces the use and existence of that side of the body.
- Dress/undress one-half of the body at a time: do the top half first then the bottom half. DO NOT dress by putting underwear on first and other clothes second; the patient will become fatigued by having to stand several times.
- Let the person do as much as possible without becoming frustrated, and ensure that spasticity does not increase.
- Anyone who has difficulty getting dressed, or who needs assistance to get dressed, should avoid tight fitting clothes. It is better to buy clothes slightly bigger or to choose looser styles.
- It may be possible to reduce the number of clothes worn. For example, some women stop wearing bras or slips. Corsets are extremely difficult to put on and can be uncomfortable to wear if sitting for long periods.
- Clothes made from cotton and natural fibres are best for someone who spends much of the time sitting. They are also easier for the carer to launder.

Dressing aids are available: for example, button hooks, dressing sticks, long handled reachers, sock aids, long handled shoe horns, and elastic shoe laces.

However, dressing aids should be used with care (particularly in patients who have perceptual problems), as they can be difficult to use. Regular practice is needed – not just a one-off session.

For those who have problems with buttons, velcro can be used instead. Buttons can also be put on elastic instead of thread to make them more flexible.

For people with perceptual/visual problems, coloured thread can be used to identify the side of the garment more easily. For example, using red thread around the arm holes for the affected side.

Someone may manage a task if they are given prompting or help to start. Avoid doing everything for them: for example, do one button to help someone line up the rest of the buttons; help with the affected arm and let them do the rest.

Whether the patient is able to dress themself, or if they need assistance, the rule is to dress the affected side first and undress it last. This method protects the affected side and guards against damage to the shoulder which is vulnerable. It also ensures that dressing is carried out in a controlled manner.

Vests and jumpers

It is best to lay the garment out on the patient's lap or in front of them on a bed, with the back facing upwards. The affected arm is put in first. Work as much of the material as possible over the elbow to prevent the sleeve falling down at the next stage. When the arm is in, work the other arm into the other sleeve. Finally, use the non-affected hand to grip the back of the vest and pull it over the head.

Pants and trousers

The affected leg is again dressed first. If the patient has problems bending but feels able to dress themself, a long handled pick-up stick can be used to thread the garment onto the foot. Alternatively, a low footstool may be used to raise the feet. Again ensure that the leg is in the garment as far as possible. Next put the non-affected leg in. If the patient has poor standing, they should get both pants and trousers up to the mid thigh and stand once only to pull both garments up. If standing is very poor, it is possible with practice for carers to do a 'bottom' wash and dry and whisk clothes up in one stand. Some male patients find wearing braces a useful way of getting the trousers up. Patients should never stand in socks or stockings unless there is carpet on the floor – it is very easy to slip. If the patient is nervous of bending forward, it is useful initially to have the therapist or carer sitting in front of them. If patients have very poor standing balance, or have a frail carer, they may be encouraged to put trousers on while lying on the bed.

Other garments

Socks, tights and stockings   Special aids such as stocking/sock aids and tight aids can be purchased. However, many patients who have had a stroke find these difficult to use. Check if it is possible to try such items out before purchasing.

Bras   These are often difficult for patients to put on, and it may be best to buy some front fastening bras. If this is not possible, or the patient is reluctant to change, they can fasten the bra at the front around the waist, spin it round and put the arms in. There are also bras available which have no fastenings and which can be pulled over the head.

Neckties   Clip on ties can now be purchased which save having to tie a knot. Otherwise, recommend that ties are not completely loosened after being worn, and re-use the knot.

Shoes   These again can be a problem to put on, especially if the patient has to wear a splint. Aids such as elastic shoe laces, long-handled shoe horns and long-handled pick-up sticks can be valuable. There is a method of tying shoe laces using one hand, but it is quite difficult to learn and requires much practice.

Undressing

For undressing the technique is always reversed. Clothing on the unaffected arm is removed first and the affected last. For the lower limb, one stand can be used to pull down all lower garments and then sit to remove over legs and feet. The OT teaching the patient to get dressed may often begin by practising undressing, as this is always easier. In some instances patients learn to undress completely before progressing on to dressing.

Cooking and domestic tasks

For patients living at home, there is a real danger of wrapping people who have had a stroke 'in cotton wool'. It is important that they still feel useful and able to contribute to the household chores. If they are able to do some light dusting or cleaning around the house, encourage this – even if the ornaments for dusting have to be brought to them.

Carers should take as much help from others as possible: for example, by getting the shopping delivered, letting friends help with the washing or hoovering. A home help may assist with the more strenuous jobs around the house.

With regard to the kitchen, many one-handed gadgets are available which enable the patient to carry out tasks such as peeling vegetables, whisking food, opening tins. It is a good idea to get someone to practice making themself (and you!) a hot drink.

General advice:

- Everything should be accessible in the kitchen; tea kept in a high cupboard or milk in a low fridge may be difficult to reach.
- Where possible, group items together: for example, have mugs, tea, sugar,

milk and biscuits in the same area to avoid the patient and/or carer having to move backwards and forwards across the kitchen.

- Recommend the purchase of a kettle which switches itself off.
- If the patient tires easily, a perching stool with a backrest may be beneficial.
- Kitchen trolleys are very useful, as they can be used to assist walking and to transport objects around the kitchen and into another room.
- Bags can be clipped onto frames to transport small objects.
- Local resource centres are useful for seeing what is available and for experimenting with gadgets on the market.

If the patient is unable to cook or make him/herself a hot drink safely, a flask of tea or coffee can be provided for when they are alone. The liquid should not be too hot nor the flask lid put on too tight. However, if carers are worried about doing this, they could ask a friend or neighbour to pop in while they are out.

Getting around outside

Getting out of the house is important, not just for a change of air or a change of scenery, but because of the achievement in itself. However, there can be many physical barriers which may it difficult for disabled people and their carers to get out and about. These barriers can be anything from steps and uneven surfaces to high kerbs and even other people. Some local councils publish helpful leaflets and guides which give information on access to public buildings and local facilities.

An important consideration must be whether the patient needs a wheelchair or not as someone who is mobile around the house may still have problems when it comes to walking down the high street. Some patients refuse to use a wheelchair because they do not want to be considered disabled. If that is so, then their opinion must be respected. If a wheelchair is needed for holidays or special days out, it may be loaned from the Red Cross or from some other voluntary agencies. Local Disablement Service Centres provide wheelchairs for more long-term use.

General tips:

- Self-propelling wheelchairs with two large back wheels and two small front ones are easier to use in getting up and down kerbs and steps. Wheelchairs with four small wheels (transit wheelchairs) are often given to carers.
- Check that the tyres are properly inflated; wheelchairs with flat tyres are hard to push.
- Check that the brakes are working and get the patient into the habit of ensuring the brakes are put on when the wheelchair is stopped. An extra long brake lever can be provided for ease of use by a disabled person.
- Check that arm rests are correctly fitted.
- Ensure that there are two foot rests and that these are locked in place. The height of the foot rests is important and should be adjusted so that neither the hips, knees or ankles of the patient are bent more than 90°.

- If the wheelchair is used regularly, a cushion should be used. Special cushions for those with pressure sores (or potential pressure sores) are available from the Disablement Services Centre.
- If the carer is frail, or the local area is hilly, it is possible to get a powered wheelchair.

Driving

Probably the most important thing to say about driving is that it is a legal requirement for someone who has a stroke to inform the DVLA (Driver and Vehicle Licensing Agency). All patients who have had a stroke may not drive for one month. If the patient's GP says that it is all right to drive after this time, they should check with their insurers to confirm they are still covered.

- Research has been carried out to enable predictions to be made about driving performance on the basis of mental ability and reaction time (Nouri & Lincoln, 1992). This test is now commercially available from Nottingham Ltd., 17 Ludlow Hill Road, West Bridgeford, Notts.
- Patients who are worried about resuming driving, or who have lost confidence, can go out with a driving instructor in a dual-controlled car to assess any difficulties.
- An automatic car may be easier to drive than one with gears, but encourage patients to try out one before buying.
- Modifications such as steering aids, left foot accelerators and rotating car seats (for ease of getting in and out of the car) are available. However, assessment and practice is important; patients can be referred to specialist driving centres by their GP for assessment and help.
- Some motoring organizations have special services for disabled drivers.
- If the patient is not able to drive after their stroke, transport is an important consideration. The carer may not feel able to take a driving test if they have never driven before. Explore local schemes, such as Dial-a-ride, enlist the help of friends and family and, if the budget permits, use a taxi (always say if a wheelchair needs to be transported when ordering).
- The orange badge scheme (operated by social services) allows disabled people to park near shops and entertainment.
- A useful leaflet *Driving after Stroke* is available from the Stroke Association.

Leisure

Boredom is a problem which has not always merited the attention it deserves, yet it can lead to frustration, low mood and lack of self-worth. A survey in Nottingham found that many patients who had had a stroke were doing very few leisure activities one year after their stroke (Drummond, 1990). It is very important that people continue former hobbies or find new ones in order to have a sense of purpose in life. Some people do not want to continue to do a hobby they have done all their life if they cannot do it so well. Others are just happy to continue former pursuits regardless of the standard they achieve. Everyone is different and will want to pursue different hobbies.

- Consider local resources: local libraries may stock large print books, tapes or videos; membership of a video club may make watching television more purposeful; local leisure centres may have special groups for the disabled such as swimming groups; local colleges may run classes which would be of interest – for example, flower arranging, music appreciation; churches or halls may run social and luncheon clubs.
- Some patients need special equipment to enable them to carry out activities. Local Disabled Living Centres can be useful in identifying and trying out equipment that may be useful: for example, playing card holders, sticky mats to hold puzzles, extra large puzzles, long-handled tools for the garden. Some of this equipment may be relatively expensive, so it is worthwhile for the patient to try it out first and then drop hints at birthdays and other present giving times.
- Specific charities and organizations can provide specialist information and help. For example, the Stroke Association and ADA can provide information on stroke groups, and various charities can give advice on holidays. Some specialist organizations can offer specific advice for the disabled: for example, on photography, golf, or fishing.
- Do not overlook the obvious ways in which people spend spare time such as reading newspapers and magazines, and watching the television. Watching TV as a hobby is fine as long as it is purposeful and does not just provide noise in the background. Getting out of the house to go to the park, going out for lunch, or meeting up with friends in the pub are also valuable ways of spending time.
- Hobbies can be shared between the carer and stroke patient or they can provide the carer with valuable time to pursue their own interests.
- There is evidence that leisure participation is related to psychological well-being (Drummond & Walker, 1996; Parker *et al.*, 1997).

General advice for carers

The role of carer can be a difficult, demanding and physically exhausting one. The following general advice should be offered to those in such a position:

(1) Let the person who has had a stroke do as much as possible for him/herself within their physical capabilities. This not only encourages them to do more and builds up their self-confidence, but it also relieves the burden on you. The more that you do, the more dependent you will make the patient and

the more work you will create for yourself. A good example of this is dressing: often carers are reluctant to watch someone struggle to put on their clothes or become exasperated because the process takes so long, so they then intervene and help the person get dressed. Unfortunately, lack of practice means that the patient may lose the ability to dress altogether, and the carer is forced into the situation of helping the patient every day.

(2)   It is very easy to fall into the trap of treating someone who needs help with many everyday tasks as though they were a child. It is important not to do this, as it undermines the patient's confidence. Instead try to offer encouragement and praise which is constructive and not patronising.

(3)   Accept help! Do not try to do everything yourself. Take advantage of friends or relatives who offer practical help with housework or shopping. If you need to help the patient with some activities, you have already increased your volume of work – so don't struggle on. Remember, you are of little use to the patient if you are constantly exhausted.

(4)   Ask for help. Many carers feel that it is an admission of failure to ask for information or help – this is *not* true. If you have particular problems, seek professional help and ensure you are getting all the financial benefits to which you are entitled.

(5)   Everyone needs time to pursue their own hobbies and interests. Allow time to do this from the beginning and take some time every week to do something enjoyable. If you are concerned about leaving the patient, try and think about possible solutions: can you put the telephone beside him/her; leave a snack and hot drink; arrange for someone to call in; is there a Crossroads Scheme or volunteer agency in your area which could help (see Appendix for Crossroads Case Scheme address)? Remember also that it may be just as important for the patient to have time without you as for you to have time without them.

Assessment by an OT

All occupational therapists should carry out regular assessments of their patients in order to monitor progress and to evaluate the effects of treatment. The vital point to stress is that the assessments used must be both valid (that is, measure what they are meant to be measuring) and reliable (give the same result under the same conditions). There are many assessments from which to choose, so therapists should not make the mistake of spending time trying to devise their own scale when full-time researchers have been working on these for years.

With regard to ADL scales, possible choices for patients who have had a stroke include: the Barthel Index (Collin *et al.*, 1988); the Rivermead ADL Scale (Lincoln & Edmans, 1990); or the Nottingham Extended ADL Scale (Nouri & Lincoln, 1987). There are, of course, disadvantages to all of these. The most common criticism made of such scales by OTs is that they are insensitive to small changes in performance and often have a floor or ceiling effect (that is, are unable to discriminate between those with either very poor or very good performance). Whilst this may be true, such scales are still better than using no assessment at all and they do provide reliable and valid information.

There are many other general areas which the OT may need to assess including motor function, perceptual performance, mood and depression, as well as more specific areas such as neglect, driving, work performance and leisure participation. A list of possible assessments which may be used is contained in Table 11.1 (readers are also directed to an excellent book by Wade (1992) which lists many tools and provides valuable comments about their use).

Table 11.1   Possible assessment tools.

Area of assessment	Possible tool	Author(s)
Motor function	Rivermead Motor Assessment	Lincoln & Leadbitter (1979)
Perceptual performance	Rivermead Perceptual Assessment Battery	Whiting *et al.* (1985); *see* also Siev & Freishtat (1976)
Mood	General Health Questionnaire	Goldberg & Hillier (1979)
Depression	Wakefield Depression Inventory	Snaith *et al.* (1971)

References

Andrews, K. (1984) What would occupational therapists do if they had more staff? *International Rehabilitation Medicine* **7**, 137–9.

Collin, C., Wade, D.T., Davis, S. & Horne, V. (1988) The Barthel ADL Index: a reliability study. *International Disability Studies* **10**, 61–3.

Drummond, A.E.R. (1990) Leisure activity after stroke. *International Disability Studies* **12**, 157–60.

Drummond, A.E.R. & Walker, M.F. (1996) Generalisation of the effects of leisure rehabilitation for stroke patients. *British Journal of Occupational Therapy* **59**, 330–34.

Ebrahim, S. & Nouri, F.M. (1987) Caring for stroke patients at home. *International Rehabilitation Medicine* **8**, 171–3.

Goldberg, D.P. & Hillier, V.F. (1979) A scaled version of the General Health Questionnaire. *Psychological Medicine* **9**, 139–45.

Hopson, S. (1981) The principles of activities of daily living. In *The Practice of Occupational Therapy*. An introduction to the treatment of physical dysfunction (Turner, A., ed.). Churchill Livingstone, London.

Lincoln, N.B. & Edmans, J.A. (1990) A re-validation of the Rivermead ADL scale for elderly stroke patients. *Age and Ageing* **19**, 19–24.

Lincoln, N.B. & Leadbitter, D. (1979) Assessment of motor function in stroke patients. *Physiotherapy* **68**, 48–51.

Nouri, F.M. & Lincoln, N.B. (1987) An extended ADL scale for use with stroke patients. *Clinical Rehabilitation* **1**, 301–5.

Nouri, F.M. & Lincoln, N.B. (1992) Validation of a cognitive assessment: predicting driving performance after stroke. *Clinical Rehabilitation* **6**, 275–81.

Parker, C.J., Gladman, J.R.F. & Drummond, A.E.R. (1997) The role of leisure in stroke rehabilitation. *Disability and Rehabilitation* **19**, 1–5.

Siev, E. & Freishtat, B. (1976) *Perceptual Dysfunction in the Adult Stroke Patient: A Manual for Evaluation and Treatment*. Slack Inc., New Jersey.

Smith, S. (1989) How occupational therapy staff spend their work time. *British Journal of Occupational Therapy* **52**(3), 82–7.

Snaith, R.P., Ahmed, S.N., Mehta, S. & Hamilton, M. (1971) Assessment of the severity of primary depressive illness: Wakefield self-assessment depression inventory. *Psychological Medicine* **1**, 143–9.

Stroke Association (1992) *How occupational therapy helps stroke patients*. Stroke Association, CHSA House, Whitecross Street, London EC1Y 8JJ.

Wade, D.T. (1992) *Measurement in Neurological Rehabilitation*. Oxford Medical Publications, Oxford.

Walker, M.F. & Lincoln, N.B. (1991) Factors affecting dressing performance after stroke. *Journal of Neurology, Neurosurgery and Psychiatry* **54**, 699–701.

Walker, M.F., Drummond, A.E.R. & Lincoln, N.B. (1996) Evaluation of dressing practice for stroke patients after discharge from hospital: a cross over design. *Clinical Rehabilitation* **10**, 23–31.

Whiting, S.E., Lincoln, N.B., Cockburn, J. & Bhavnani, G. (1985) *The Rivermead Perceptual Assessment Battery*. NFER-Nelson, Windsor.

Appendix: Organizations supporting both the individual and carers

The following lists are extensive but far from exhaustive. They were compiled with the general assistance of Action for Dysphasic Adults, Age Concern, the Stroke Association and the National Aphasia Association in the United States.

United Kingdom organizations

There are many organizations operating at a local level, and information on these is normally available in hospitals, general practitioners' waiting rooms and public libraries. The Citizens Advice Bureau is also a valuable source of information on matters relating to disability benefits and other help available. Local social service departments are responsible for community care and organize facilities such as home helps and day centres. Some local organizations have been included to illustrate the type of activity which can be provided.

Principal stroke organizations

Action for Dysphasic Adults (ADA)

Action for Dysphasic Adults is the only national organization in the UK providing a service solely for people with dysphasia and their families. It was set up by Diana Law MBE, who had suffered a severe stroke in 1967. She had had a distinguished war time career and subsequently became a senior executive in two international companies. In 1974 she proposed a system of speech clubs in the national press and six years later she founded the charity ADA. Amongst other activities, they have funded a number of research projects into various aspects of aphasia therapy, including a project on a counselling service for dysphasic patients.

The organization has made a survey of speech and language therapy services for people with dysphasia, showing that there is considerable variation in the adequacy of services available.

One of ADA's most recent projects is the development of a training package for managers, matrons and carers in residential homes. ADA also provides a series of booklets on different aspects of communication problems found in dysphasia, and it publishes a quarterly newsletter *Speaking Up*. ADA organizes study days and national conferences, and dysphasic people play an active part in these as well as having representatives on the organization's council. There are a small number of regional branches which work closely with the local speech therapy service.

Address:
1 Royal Street
London SE1 7LL
Tel: 0171-261 9572
Fax: 0171-928 9542
e-mail: ADANATION@aol.com
Web site: http://glaxocentre.merseysideorg/ada.html

Age Concern

Enables older people to solve problems themselves, by providing as much or as little
support as they need. Facilities include lunch clubs, day centres and home visiting. Their
publications include '*Caring for someone who has had a stroke*,' a highly informative and
useful book is available for purchase. Listed below are the four main Age Concern offices.

Age Concern England
1268 London Road
London SW16 4ER
Tel: 0181-679 8000

Age Concern Scotland
113 Rose Street
Edinburgh EH2 3DT
Tel: 0131-220 3345

Age Concern Cymru
4th Floor, 1 Cathedral Road
Cardiff CF1 9SD
Tel: 01222-371566
Web site: www.ace.org.uk/infopoint/

Age Concern Northern Ireland
3 Lower Crescent
Belfast BT7 1NR
Tel: 01232-245729

Aphasia Computer Team (ACT)

Initially concerned with research into the use of computers in the treatment of stroke
impaired individuals, the team have gone on to develop a range of valuable software
designed to assist the dysphasic adult in both the clinic and at home

ACT runs courses for speech and language therapists and others involved in the
rehabilitation of communication skills. Its prime software development has been INTACT
which provides over 700 graded exercises in a multimedia environment. Access can be
achieved from a switch, the space bar or the full keyboard, and the computer offers visual
clues derived from scanned photographs. Auditory clues are recorded digitally and include
both speech and environmental sounds.

Therapists can design their own exercises to suit individual needs, and considerable
support is provided by the ACT team. The patient's responses are recorded and analysed
by the computer, and those who have suitable hardware in their homes can be given tasks
to complete on their own or with family support.
Address:
Speech and Language Therapy Research Unit
Frenchay Hospital
Bristol BS16 1LE
Tel: 0117-970 1212 Ext. 2291/0117-918 6529
Fax: 0117-970 1119
e-mail: admin@speechtherapy.org.uk

Chartered Society of Physiotherapists

The professional body concerned with the training and practice of physiotherapists has set up a list for registered assistants. A specific committee is concerned with such areas as a Code of Conduct, training and terms and conditions of employment. In considering the delegation of tasks to assistants and other support workers, the society are unequivocal in stating that physiotherapists are ultimately responsible for the management of their patients and must ensure that assistants or technical instructors are trained to undertake the delegated tasks. In its guidelines for training, the society considers that 'each physiotherapy department should have an on-going training programme for helpers relevant to their roles within the service'.

Address:

14 Bedford Row
London WC1R 4ED
Tel: 0171-242 1941
Fax: 0171-306 6611

City University Dysphasic Group

As part of the university's department of language and communication science, the group provides language therapy for dysphasic adults and operates a programme of research into the linguistic, psychological and social aspects of aphasia. Both research staff and group members have been closely involved in the production of *The Aphasia Handbook* for dysphasic people, their families and carers. A major theme of the group's current approach is the encouragement of self-advocacy.

Address:

Department of Language and Communication Science
City University
Northampton Square
London EC1V OHB
Tel: 0171-477 8288
Fax: 0171 477 8577
Web site: www.city@ac.

College of Occupational Therapists

The professional body concerned with the training of occupational therapists. In its *Advice Note on Occupational Therapy Helpers*, the college states that the helper's role is to complement and provide continuity of the work of the qualified occupational therapist in aiding patients in their recovery. Helpers will be members of a multi-disciplinary team and must follow the programme of treatment and activity approved by trained professional staff. In addition, a helper must be under the over-all supervision of a trained, state registered occupational therapist and must always have access to one for advice and direction. Helpers 'must never undertake initial assessments and/or amend treatment programmes.' Occupational therapy departments may also employ technical instructors, art and music instructors and teachers of handicraft who, depending on their qualifications and experience, may work more or less independently without direct and regular supervision.

Address:
106–14 Borough High Street
London SE1 1LB
Tel: 0171-357 6480
Fax: 0171-450 2299

COMPAID Trust (Computer Aid for Speech Impaired and Disabled People)

The trust provides for the welfare, training and where possible future employment of speech impaired and disabled adults by giving advice on computer technology and by promoting its use. In addition the trust fosters the development of assessment services and research and development of software to meet specific needs. From the outset clients have included people who have suffered strokes as well as those with other neurological and physical disabilities.
Address:
Pembury Hospital
Tunbridge Wells
Kent TN2 4QJ
Tel/Fax: 01892-824 060

Different Strokes

A registered charity set up by a group of younger stroke survivors with the express aim of comprehensive support for individuals who have suffered strokes under the age of retirement. The charity provides a counselling service, information packs, special access to gyms, physiotherapy sessions and swimming. It also offers advice and information on further and higher education and job opportunities as well as information about state benefits and anti-discrimination rights.
Address:
Sir Walter Scott House
2 Broadway Market
London E8 4QJ
Tel/Fax: 0171-249 6645
e-mail: differentstrokes@demon.co.uk
Web site: www.strokes.demon.co.uk

Royal College of Speech and Language Therapists

The professional body concerned with the education, training and practice of speech and language therapists recognizes that assistants working with either children or adults require different training and expertise. A core curriculum for training has been drawn up by the Association of Speech and Language Therapy Managers, and it is planned that a National Vocational Qualification will be available. At present, the training of speech and language therapy assistants is dependent on in-service course available within the different districts.
Address:
7 Bath Place
Rivington Street
London EC2A 3SU
Tel: 0171-613 3855
Fax: 0171-613 3854
Website: www.rcslt.org

Stroke Association

The Stroke Association offers a family support scheme within the community as well as stroke clubs for families and carers of stroke patients for new stroke patients and those who live alone. The Dysphasic Support Scheme provides practical help for patients who also have communication problems.

A major aim of the association is to foster research into the causes of strokes and the means by which they may be prevented. In 1999 over 2.5 million pounds was provided for research and training from funds raised through public donations. The Dysphasic Support Scheme is in part supported by Community Services Contracts. Funds are provided to individuals in special need by means of a Welfare Grant Scheme. There are concerns that these funds are increasingly required to fill gaps in social service provision.

The extent to which Dysphasic Support volunteers work with speech therapists varies considerably, and so does the amount of training they receive. Volunteers undoubtedly provide an important supportive role in the total rehabilitation service, and the Stroke Clubs they run may be the only social outlet for the stroke patient. Family and dysphasic support does not seek to replace the skills of professional health workers, but rather to provide a complementary service. In practice, however, the latter service may be all that is available to the dysphasic patients.

The association also produces informative booklets and leaflets on various aspects of stroke as well as two quarterly publications *Stroke News* and *Look Forward* which includes materials for dysphasic patients. There is a network of information centres, and the service is organized on a regional basis.

Address:

Stroke House

123–7 Whitecross Street

London EC1Y 8JJ

Tel: 0171-560 0300

Fax: 0171-490 2686

Web site: www.stroke.org.uk

Other UK organizations

Benefits Agency

Provides advice about state benefits for people with disabilities and their carers.

(Benefit Enquiry Line:) 0800 88 22 00

British Heart Foundation

Information on all aspects of heart disease.

14 Fitzhardinge Street

London W1H 4DH

Tel: 0171-935 0185

British Red Cross
Can lend or hire home aids for disabled people. Local branches in many areas.

9 Grosvenor Crescent
London SW1X 7EJ
Tel: 0171-235 5454

Carers National Association
Information and advice for partners and families caring for an individual with a disability.
Has offices in principal UK cities.

20–25 Glasshouse Yard
London EC1A 4JS
Tel: 0171-490 8898

Continence Foundation
Advice and information in regard to incontinence problems.

The Basement
2 Doughty Street
London WC1N 2PH
Tel: 0171-404 6875

Crossroads Care
Operates a care attendant scheme for care at home.

10 Regent Place
Rugby
Warwickshire CV21 2PN
Tel: 01788 573653

DIAL UK
Information and advice for people with disabilities.

Park Lodge
St Catherine's Hospital
Tickhill Road, Balby
Doncaster DN4 8QN
Tel: 01302 310123

Disabled Living Foundation
Information about aids designed to assist a disabled person.

380–384 Harrow Road
London W9 2HU
Tel: 0171-289 6111
Web site: www.dlf.org.uk/advice/index.htm

Headway (National Head Injuries Association)

For people who are disabled physically or mentally as a result of head injury.

7 King Edward Court
King Edward Street
Nottingham NG1 1EW
Tel: 0115 912 1000

Holiday Care Service

Free information on holidays for elderly or disabled people and their carers.

2nd Fl. Imperial Buildings
Victoria Road
Horley, Surrey RH6 7PZ
Tel: 01293 771500

RADAR (Royal Association for Disability and Rehabilitation)

Information about aids and mobility, holidays, sport and leisure for disabled people.

Unit 12, City Forum
250 City Road
London EC1V 8AF
Tel: 0171-250 3222

SPOD (Association to Aid the Sexual and Personal Relationships of People with a Disability)

Telephone counselling and advice.

286 Camden Road
London N7 0BJ
Tel: 0171-607 8851

Organizations outside the UK

Australia

Australian Brain Foundation

Suite 21, Regent House
37–45 Alexander St.
Crow's Nest NSW 2065
Tel: (08) 8212 5595; Fax: (08) 8211 7517

Australian Self-Help Index

Provides listings of the major organizations offering support for the disabled.
Web site: www.accessnable.com.au/selfhelp.htm

Carers Association of Australia
Has a stroke fact sheet and other information.
Web site: www.carers.asn.au/stroke.html

National Stroke Foundation
Level 2, 394–400 Little Bourke St.
Victoria 3000, Australia
Tel: 03 9670 1000; Fax: 03 9670 9300
E-mail: admin@natstroke.asn.au
Web site: www.natstroke.asn.au

Austria

Aphasie Club
Kegelgasse 27/1
A-1030 Wien

Belgium

Association Internationale Aphasie
Avenue des Heros, 50
B-1160 Bruxelles

Coeur et Prevention
Rue de Cypres, 14
1000 Bruxelles

Canada

Association Queboise des Personnes Aphasiques
4565 Queen Mary Road
Montreal H3W 1W5
Tel: (514) 340 3540

Pat Arato Aphasia Centre
53 The Links Road
Toronto, Ontario M2P 1T7
Tel: (416) 226 3636

Stroke Survivors Support Group
L.A. Miller Centre
St John's, Newfoundland AIB 3V6
Tel: (709) 737 6560

Czech Republic

Institute of Phonetics
Jan Palachovo Nam, 2
CZ 116 38 Praha 1

Denmark

Hjerne Sagen
Henrik Ibsenvej, 44
DK-8500 Grenaa

Estonia

Eesti Afsiahit
Kaluri6-6, Haaneeme
EE-3006 Viimsi

Finland

Aivohalvaus-je afasialiirro ry
Detmarinkuja 3, E27
FIN-20610 Turku

Finnish Heart Association
Fredrikinkatu, 20B
00120 Helsinki
Tel: (90) 650 288

France

Federation Nationale des Aphasiques de France
Rue Montyon, 22
F-76610 Le Havre

French Heart Association
50 rue du Rocher
F-75008 Paris
Tel: 01 45 22 52 51

Germany

Bundesverband der Aphasiker
Robert Koch Strasse, 34
D-97080 Wurzburg

German Medical Association
Bundesartskammer
Hacdenkampstrasse 1
POB 41, 0220 Koln
N. Rhein WE 500

Gibraltar

Stroke Group
St Bernard's Hospital
Gibraltar

Greece

Association Panellenique des Aphasiques
September 3rd Street, 128
GR-10434 Athens

Ireland

Volunteer Stroke Scheme
249 Crumlin Road
Dublin 12, Eire
Tel: 00353 1 557455
Fax: 00353 1 557013

National Rehabilitation Board
25 Clyde Road,
Dublin 4, Eire
Tel: 00353-1 684181

Israel

MILBAT
Israel Centre for Technology and Accessibility
Tel-Hashomer 52621
Tel: 03-5303739

Italy

Associazone Italiana Afasici
Largo A. Gemelli, 8
I-00168 Roma

Japan

Japanese Aphasia Peer Circles
Rm 103 Heim–Tomita
2–29 Tomihia-cbo Shinjiku-ku
JAP 162 Tokyo

Stroke Research Club
Faculty of Medicine
University of Tsukuba
JAP 305 Ibaraki

Luxembourg

Association Internationale Aphasie
Um Kiem, 124A
L-8030 Strassen

Netherlands

Afasie Verenigung Nederland
Postbus 221
NL-6930 AE Westervoort

Netherland Heart Foundation
Sophialaan 10
2514 JR The Hague
Tel: 31 70 92 42 92

New Zealand

Counterstroke NZ Inc
PO Box 2320
Wellington
Tel: 04 768 487

Stroke Foundation of New Zealand
PO Box 12482
Wellington
Tel: 04 472 8099
Fax: 04 472 7019

Norway

Afasiforbundet i Norge
PB 8716 Youngstorget
N-0028 Oslo

Norske Kvinners Sanitetsforening
Postboks 5608 Briskeby
0209 Oslo 2

Poland

Polish Rehabilitation Society
'Repty' GCR Wydzia 3 Zamiejscovy
ul. Zdrojowa 6
PL 43-450
Ustron
Tel/fax: 00 48 33 54 16 32
Web site: www.gapp.pl/sol/ptreh-repty

Portugal

Associaca Natcianal de Afasicos
Rua Conde Redondo 13/5
P-1150 Lisboa

Spain

Associacio d'afasics de Catalunya
Pere Verges 1, Planta 6A
E-08020 Barcelona

Sweden

Afasiforbundet i Sverige
Kampementsgatan, 14
S-11538 Stockholm

Riksforbundet mot Hjarmans Karlsjukdomar
Wenner Gren Centre
Svcavagen 166
19tr 11346 Stockholm

Switzerland

Schweiz. Arbeitsgemeinschaft fur Aphasic
Zahringerstrasse, 19
CH-6003 Luzern

Foyer-Handicap Geneve
Links with international associations for
the disabled
http://www.foyer-handicap.ch/liensas.htm

United States

American Heart Association
Offers free and low-cost publications on strokes.
Details of local stroke support groups can be provided.

7272 Greenville Avenue
Dallas, TX 75231
Tel: (214) 373 6300 or
(800) 553 6321 – Stroke Connection Line
Website: www.americanheart.org/stroke/strokehp.htm

National Aphasia Association
Publishes a range of literature and a newsletter with details of conferences and research reports. Promotes public education and support services.

Suite 707, 156 Fifth Avenue
New York, NY 10010
Tel: (212) 255 4329 or
(800) 922 4622 – Response Centre
Web site: www.aphasia.org

National Institute of Neurological Disorders and Stroke
Provides a wide range of information and promotes research (budget for 1999 is $96,251,000).

National Institutes of Health
1, Communication Avenue
Bethesda, MD 20892-3456
Tel: (0800) 241 1044
Web site: www.ninds.nih.gov./healinfo/disorder/stroke/strokehp.htm

National Stroke Association
Offers free and low-cost publications and provides information on local support groups.

Suite I
96 Inverness Drive East
Englewood CO 80112-5112
Tel: (800) 787 6537
Web site: www.stroke.org

West Indies

W.I. Stroke Association
PO Box 449
Castries, St Lucia
Tel: 809 452 6476

Zimbabwe

Stroke Support Group
The Rotaract Club of Harare West
PO Box A 356
Avondale, Harare

Further Reading

Parr, S., Pound, C., Byng, S. & Long, B. (1999) *The Aphasia Handbook.* Connect Press, London.

Clarke, M. (1998) *Less Words More Respect: My Experience with Dysphasia.* Action for Dysphasic Adults, London.

Edelman, G. & Greenwood, R. *Jumbly Words, and Rights Where Wrongs Should Be: The Experience of Aphasia From The Inside.* Far Communications, Leicester.

Law, D. & Paterson, B. (1980) *Living After A Stroke.* Souvenir Press, London.

Lyon, J. (1998) *Coping with Aphasia.* Singular Publishing Group, San Diego, CA.

Newborn, B. (1997) *Return to Ithaca.* Penguin, New Jersey.

Parr, S., Byng, S., Gilpin, S. & Ireland, C. (1997) *Talking about Aphasia.* Open University Press, Milton Keynes.

Index